PSYCHIATRIC ASPECTS OF GENERAL PATIENT CARE

3rd Edition

By
Bonnie Fossett, MSEd, RN, CS
and
Marlene Nadler-Moodie, MSN, RN, CS

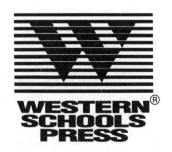

**WESTERN®
SCHOOLS
PRESS**

21 Bristol Drive
South Easton, MA 02375
1-800-618-1670

Copy Editor: Barbara Halliburton, PhD

Indexer: Sylvia Coates

Typesetter: Kathy Johnson

Library of Congress Catalog Card Number: 94-60363

Western Schools courses are designed to provide Nursing professionals with the Educational information they need to enhance their career development. The information provided within these course materials is the result of research and consultation with prominent Nursing and Medical authorities and is, to the best of our knowledge, current and accurate. However, the courses and course materials are provided with the understanding that Western Schools is not engaged in offering legal, nursing, medical, or other professional advice.

Western Schools courses and course materials are not meant to act as a substitute for seeking out professional advice or conducting individual research. When applying the information provided in the courses and course materials to individual circumstances, all recommendations must be considered in light of the uniqueness pertaining to each situation.

Western Schools course materials are intended solely for *your* use, and *not* for the benefit of providing advice or recommendations to third parties. Western Schools devoids itself of any responsibility for adverse consequences resulting from the failure to seek nursing, medical or other professional advice. Western Schools further devoids itself of any responsibility for updating or revising any programs or publications presented, published, distributed or sponsored by Western Schools unless otherwise agreed to as part of an individual purchase contract.

ISBN: 1-878025-92-9

ABOUT THE AUTHORS

Bonnie Fossett, MSEd, RN, CS, is currently Vice President of United Health Resources in charge of the continuing nursing education division; and is also the Director of Quality Systems at Portsmouth Regional Hospital and Pavilion in Portsmouth, NH. She is certified by the ANA as a Clinical Specialist in Adult Psychiatric and Mental Health Nursing, and as a Certified Professional in Healthcare Quality through the National Association for Healthcare Quality.

Marlene Nadler-Moodie, RN, MSN, CS, is currently in private practice in psychiatric and mental health nursing. She also is a curriculum developer and instructor for the University of California, San Diego Extension.

Sue Green, RN, CS, MSW, is director of patient care at St. Luke's Episcopal Hospital in Houston, Texas. She has published material on the effects of transition on work groups and mentoring nursing research.

Nancy Morgan Andreola, RN, has been a psychiatric and mental health nurse in both inpatient and community settings for 12 years. She is currently a free-lance writer and editor on medical and nursing issues and is a contributing editor at *Nursing Spectrum* magazine. She is also a crisis case manager at Mid-Bergen Community Mental Health Center in Paramus, New Jersey.

Kathy Templin, RN, MS, CCRN, has 22 years of experience working in a clinical setting. She is currently a clinical nurse specialist, MICU/CCU, at the Veterans Affairs Medical Center in La Jolla, California.

ABOUT THE SUBJECT MATTER EXPERTS

Ann Robinette, RN, MS, has 20 years of experience in psychiatric nursing and is currently a psychiatric liaison clinical nurse specialist at Pacific Presbyterian Hospital of Pacific Medical Center, San Francisco, California.

Gabriella Gerardi, RN, MA, has her master's degree is in counselor education. She is currently a nurse clinician at St. Luke's Episcopal Hospital in Houston, Texas.

Patricia Barron, MS, RN, C, is currently in private practice in psychotherapy. She is a psychiatric nurse at Hackensack Medical Center in Hackensack, New Jersey.

Vicki DeBaca, MSN, RN, has many years of experience in the health care field. She has worked in intensive care, surgery, medical/surgical units, and home health nursing. In addition, Vicki has extensive experience in the field of continuing education, providing both seminars and home-study programs. Vicki has written on a variety of topics in nursing and has had articles published in J*ONA, AJN, RN,* and *Hospital Topics.*

Portions of the following publications are reprinted with the express permission of their publishers:

1. Jacobs, J. W., Bernhard, M. R., Delgado, A., & Strain, J. J. Screening for Organic Mental Syndromes in the Medically Ill. *Annals of Internal Medicine,* 86(1), 40–45, 1977. Philadelphia, Pennsylvania.

2. *Diagnostic and Statistical Manual of Mental Disorders,* 4th ed. American Psychiatric Association. Washington DC, 1994.

3. Townsend, M. C. *Nursing Diagnoses in Psychiatric Nursing: A Pocket Guide for Care Plan Construction.* F.A. Davis Co., Philadelphia, Pennsylvania.

4. The Nurse-Client Manipulation Cycle. *Psychosocial Nursing and Mental Health Services,* SLACK, Inc. 1991.

5. Continuum of Social Responses. In *Principles and Practice of Psychiatric Nursing.* Mosby Year Book, St. Louis, Missouri, 1991.

IMPORTANT: Read these instructions *BEFORE* proceeding!

Enclosed with your course book you will find the FasTrax® answer sheet. Use this form to answer all the final exam questions that appear in this course book. If you are completing more than one course, be sure to write your answers on the appropriate answer sheet. Full instructions and complete grading details are printed on the FasTrax instruction sheet, also enclosed with your order. Please review them before starting. *If you are mailing your answer sheet(s) to Western Schools, we recommend you make a copy as a backup.*

ABOUT THIS COURSE

A "Pretest" is provided with each course to test your current knowledge base regarding the subject matter contained within this course. Your "Final Exam" is a multiple choice examination. **You will find the exam questions at the end of each chapter.** Some smaller hour courses include the exam at the end of the book.

In the event the course has less than 100 questions, mark your answers to the questions in the course book and leave the remaining answer boxes on the FasTrax answer sheet blank. **Use a black pen to fill in your answer sheet.**

A PASSING SCORE

You must score 70% or better in order to pass this course and receive your Certificate of Completion. Should you fail to achieve the required score, we will send you an additional FasTrax answer sheet so that you may make a second attempt to pass the course. Western Schools will allow you three chances to pass the same course...*at no extra charge!* After three failed attempts to pass the same course, your file will be closed.

RECORDING YOUR HOURS

Please monitor the time it takes to complete this course using the handy log sheet on the other side of this page. See below for transferring study hours to the course evaluation.

COURSE EVALUATIONS

In this course book you will find a short evaluation about the course you are soon to complete. This information is vital to providing the school with feedback on this course. The course evaluation answer section is in the lower right hand corner of the FasTrax answer sheet marked "Evaluation" with answers marked 1–25. Your answers are important to us, please take five minutes to complete the evaluation.

On the back of the FasTrax instruction sheet there is additional space to make any comments about the course, the school, and suggested new curriculum. Please mail the FasTrax instruction sheet, with your comments, back to Western Schools in the envelope provided with your course order.

TRANSFERRING STUDY TIME

Upon completion of the course, transfer the total study time from your log sheet to question #25 in the Course Evaluation. The answers will be in ranges, please choose the proper hour range that best represents your study time. You MUST log your study time under question #25 on the course evaluation.

EXTENSIONS

You have 2 years from the date of enrollment to complete this course. A six (6) month extension may be purchased. If after 30 months from the original enrollment date you do not complete the course, *your file will be closed and no certificate can be issued.*

CHANGE OF ADDRESS?

In the event you have moved during the completion of this course please call our student services department at 1-800-618-1670 and we will update your file.

A GUARANTEE YOU'LL GIVE HIGH HONORS TO

If any continuing education course fails to meet your expectations or if you are not satisfied in any manner, for any reason, you may return it for an exchange or a refund (less shipping and handling) within 30 days. Software, video and audio courses must be returned unopened.

Thank you for enrolling at Western Schools!

WESTERN SCHOOLS
P.O. Box 1930
Brockton, MA 02303
(800) 618-1670

Psychiatric Aspects of General Patient Care

WESTERN SCHOOLS PRESS

21 Bristol Drive
South Easton, MA 02375

Please use this log to total the number of hours you spend reading the text and taking the final examination (use 50-min hours).

Date	Hours Spent
——————	——————
——————	——————
——————	——————
——————	——————
——————	——————
——————	——————
——————	——————
——————	——————
——————	——————
——————	——————
——————	——————
——————	——————
——————	——————
——————	——————

TOTAL [   ]

Please log your study hours with submission of your final exam. To log your study time, fill in the appropriate circle under question 25 of the FasTrax® answer sheet under the "Evaluation" section.

PLEASE LOG YOUR STUDY HOURS WITH SUBMISSION OF YOUR FINAL EXAM. Please choose which best represents the total study hours it took to complete this 30 hour course.

A. less than 25 hours   C. 29–32 hours

B. 25–28 hours   D. greater than 32 hours

Psychiatric Aspects of General Patient Care

WESTERN SCHOOLS' NURSING
CONTINUING EDUCATION EVALUATION

Instructions: Mark your answers to the following questions with a black pen on the "Evaluation" section of your FasTrax® answer sheet provided with this course. You should not return this sheet. Please use the scale below to rate the following statements:

A	Agree Strongly	C	Disagree Somewhat
B	Agree Somewhat	D	Disagree Strongly

The course content met the following education objectives:

1. Identifies the major components of the communication process.

2. Illustrates the differences between assessment tools and identifies their components.

3. Indicates how the concept of anxiety relates to the nursing care of patients.

4. Identifies affective illness and how principles of psychiatric nursing affect care of the patient.

5. Illustrates how to assess suicidal ideation in patients.

6. Illustrates how to recognize psychosis.

7. Identifies the chemically dependent and impaired patient.

8. Identifies the signs and symptoms of confusion in a patient.

9. Identifies the manifestations of anorexia nervosa and bulimia.

10. Describes nursing interventions that can be used to manage a violent patient.

11. Identifies interventions to decrease noncompliance.

12. Identifies manipulative behaviors and discusses appropriate nursing interventions.

13. Discusses common psychological responses to acute cardiac illness.

14. Identifies psychotropic medications and discusses medication administration.

15. Discusses ethical and legal issues that are of concern in the practice of mental health nursing.

16. This offering met my professional education needs.

17. The objectives met the overall purpose/goal of the course.

18. The course was generally well written and the subject matter explained thoroughly. (If no please explain on the back of the FasTrax instruction sheet.)

19. The content of this course was appropriate for home study.

20. The final examination was well written and at an appropriate level for the content of the course.

Please complete the following research questions in order to help us better meet your educational needs. Pick the ONE answer which is most appropriate.

21. What was the SINGLE most important reason you chose this course?

    A. Low Price

    B. New or Newly revised course

    C. High interest/Required course topic

    D. Number of Contact Hours Needed

22. Where do you work? (If your place of employment is not listed below, please leave this question blank.)

    A. Hospital

    B. Medical Clinic/Group Practice/ HMO/Office setting

    C. Long Term Care/Rehabilitation Facility/Nursing Home

    D. Home Health Care Agency

23. Which field do you specialize in?

    A. Medical/Surgical

    B. Geriatrics

    C. Pediatrics/Neonatal

    D. Other

24. For your last renewal, how many months BEFORE your license expiration date did you order your course materials?

    A. 1–3 months

    B. 4–6 months

    C. 7–12 months

    D. Greater than 12 months

25. **PLEASE LOG YOUR STUDY HOURS WITH SUBMISSION OF YOUR FINAL EXAM.** Please choose which best represents the total study hours it took to complete this 30 hour course.

    A. less than 25 hours

    B. 25–28 hours

    C. 29–32 hours

    D. greater than 32 hours

CONTENTS

PRETEST

PSYCHIATRIC ASPECTS OF GENERAL PATIENT CARE

Begin by taking the pretest. Compare your answers on the pretest to the answer key (located in the back of the book). Circle those test items that you missed. The pretest answer key indicates the course chapters where the content of that question is discussed.

Next, read each chapter. Focus special attention on the chapters where you made incorrect answer choices. Exam questions are provided at the end of each chapter so that you can assess your progress and understanding of the material.

1. The process of communication is best characterized as:

   a. Stationary
   b. Multidimensional
   c. Motivational
   d. Ongoing

2. Which of the following is a psychiatric nurse's best therapeutic tool?

   a. Sphygmomanometer
   b. Good language skills
   c. Method of observation
   d. Herself or himself

3. Assessing a patient is important because it allows the nurse to do which of the following?

   a. Report and document.
   b. Provide support and reassurance.
   c. Complete charting requirements.
   d. Determine the patient's problem and plan interventions.

4. NANDA is the acronym for which of the following?

   a. North American Nursing Diagnosis Association
   b. National Action for Nursing Diagnosis in America
   c. National Association for Nursing Diagnosis in America
   d. North American National Diagnostic Action

5. A threat to a person's self-esteem can do which of the following?

   a. Make the person sick.
   b. Be an event.
   c. Precipitate a major nervous breakdown.
   d. Cause anxiety.

6. Which of the following are physiologic responses to anxiety?

   a. Memory impairment, queasiness
   b. Choking, fatigue
   c. Restlessness, palpitations
   d. Chest pain, decreased pulse rate

7. Establishing trust, maintaining a calm demeanor, and acting in a nonthreatening manner are appropriate nursing interventions for a patient who is which of the following?

    a. Critically ill

    b. Anorectic

    c. Hard of hearing

    d. Anxious

8. Fear, ineffective coping, and deficit self-care are all nursing diagnoses for patients who have which of the following?

    a. Depression

    b. Psychosis

    c. Personality disorder

    d. Anxiety

9. Bipolar affective illness is which of the following?

    a. A life-threatening illness

    b. Baby blues

    c. An affective illness with bouts of highs and lows

    d. A reactive depression

10. Murder turned inward refers to which of the following?

    a. Rage

    b. A violent assault

    c. A causative theory of suicide

    d. An untoward incident

11. What nursing intervention is most important when working with a suicidal patient?

    a. Provide support and reassurance.

    b. Teach stress management.

    c. Change the patient's wound dressing.

    d. Create a safe environment.

12. What is the definition of echolalia?

    a. Repetition of what someone else says

    b. Repetition of one's own words

    c. A catatonic stupor

    d. Psychosis

13. Which of the following is characterized by dysphoric mood; vivid, unpleasant dreams; and an increase in appetite?

    a. Heroin use

    b. Suicidal ideation

    c. Cocaine withdrawal

    d. Anorexia nervosa

14. What are the two commonly used medications for alcohol withdrawal?

    a. Chlordiazepoxide and pentobarbital

    b. Diazepam and triazolam

    c. Chlordiazepoxide and lorazepam

    d. Alcohol and phenobarbital

15. The signs and symptoms of heroin overdose include which of the following?

    a. Decreased respirations, pinpoint pupils, pulmonary edema

    b. Depression, fatigue, pinpoint pupils

    c. Shock, increased blood pressure, insomnia

    d. Pinpoint pupils, decreased respiration, mouth sores

16. A metabolic disturbance, substance abuse, and injury are all problems that can precipitate which of the following psychiatric conditions?

    a. Schizophrenia

    b. Confusion

    c. Schizoaffective illness

    d. Alzheimer's disease

17. Which of the following considerations should be given priority in the management of a confused 86-year-old woman?

    a. Hygiene

    b. Hearing

    c. Safety

    d. Privacy

18. A nursing diagnosis of disturbance in body image is indicative of which of the following disorders?

    a. Organic brain disorder

    b. Nutritional disorder

    c. Personality disorder

    d. Eating disorder

19. Defusing an incident is the best way to manage which of the following types of patients?

    a. A violent patient

    b. A patient who has an organic brain syndrome

    c. A hysterical patient

    d. A catatonic patient

20. Which of the following is an environmental risk factor associated with noncompliance?

    a. Number of health care providers

    b. Limited income

    c. Credentials of care provider

    d. On-the-job support system

21. Which of the following is a defining characteristic of a competent patient?

    a. The patient has not been coerced into making a decision.

    b. The patient makes the right decisions for his or her health care situation.

    c. The patient is oriented and alert.

    d. The patient is physically and mentally able to participate in making decisions.

22. According to the objective criteria for a nursing assessment of manipulation, which of the following scenarios describes a manipulative patient?

    a. At 10:45 a.m., for the second time, Mr. J. approaches the nurse's station for his 10 a.m. medications.

    b. The nurse observes Mr. B. hiding his medication under his pillow. He denies having done it and reminds her that he is the King of France.

    c. The nurse finds a bottle of whiskey in Ms. M.'s drawer. Ms. M. immediately admits to having hidden it there and is genuinely remorseful.

    d. Knowing that an important radiograph was scheduled for today, Mr. M. leaves the unit. He laughs when, on his return, the nurse reminds him that it is against policy to leave the hospital without informing the staff and that he missed a very important test.

23. Antipsychotics are used to treat which of the following?

    a. Toxic reactions and hiccoughs

    b. Delusions and hallucinations

    c. Depression

    d. Extrapyramidal side effects

24. Which of the following are both anxiolytics?

    a. Clonazepam and Clozaril

    b. Temazepam and diazepam

    c. Haldol and amobarbital

    d. Xanax and Valium

25. Which of the following is the legal concern addressed in the Tarasoff decision?

    a. Informed consent versus right to life

    b. Competency versus commitment

    c. Duty to warn versus confidentiality

    d. Privilege versus confidentiality

PREFACE

In general, nurses understand the importance of maintaining and updating the skills needed to care for patients who have emotional problems and mental illness. A basic premise is that all patients who are being cared for by health professionals are undergoing some emotional trials; the patient may be anxious, have a serious illness, or be in pain or worse. Even the joyful occasion of giving birth is a highly stressful event that may be associated with some emotional sequelae.

Patients who are undergoing emotional situations or crises require care that goes beyond the basic medical regimen. Often it is the nurse's responsibility to deal with these problems in patients because he or she spends more time at the bedside than any other health care provider.

Some patients who have a frank psychiatric illness or a history of one may require hospitalization. Some patients with no previous psychiatric problems may experience emotional problems when they are hospitalized. A patient may need hospitalization because of an exacerbation of a psychiatric illness or its sequelae, such as sometimes occurs in people who are unsuccessful with a suicide attempt. Also, psychiatric patients may experience illness or injury; they may break a leg, have a cardiac problem, or have cancer, to name a few situations. In any event, the care of patients who have psychiatric illness and of those who are undergoing emotional crises poses an increased challenge to nursing.

CHAPTER 1

THE COMMUNICATION PROCESS AND INTERPERSONAL SKILLS

CHAPTER OBJECTIVE

After completing this chapter, the reader will be able to recognize major components of the communication process and specify which interpersonal skills are needed to ensure good nursing care.

LEARNING OBJECTIVES

After studying this chapter, the reader will be able to

1. Recognize the basic components of the communication process.

2. Specify which components can improve interpersonal skills.

3. Indicate two strategies that are used to make communication more effective.

4. Select at least three helpful phrases for good communication.

5. Choose three phrases that might close off effective communication.

6. Recognize barriers to communication.

COMMUNICATION

Communication is at the core of psychiatric nursing. Eliciting information about the feelings, events, views, and thoughts of the patient is of the utmost importance. Simultaneously, being responsive to patients and establishing a rapport will facilitate patients' ability to better understand their emotions and cope with their own reactions.

Process

Communication is an ongoing process. Dynamic in nature, it flows, bends, expands, and contracts in both verbal and nonverbal forms. It often takes the form of written words, pictures, signs, and graphic advertisements. Yet, spoken words may or may not be used. What is not being said may be just as important as what is said. Body language plays an important role, because through gestures and facial expressions we communicate nonverbally.

Most of us are most comfortable with communicating by speaking. Our language, tone of voice, expressions, and word usage need to be clear, and we should get feedback to make sure we have been understood correctly.

Components

Three basic components are needed for communication to occur:

1. Sender
2. Message
3. Receiver

Briefly stated, the sender delivers the message to the receiver. A simple example is the question nurses ask every day: "How are you feeling?"

The sender is the nurse.

The message is the question, "How are you feeling?"

The receiver is the patient.

Nonverbal communication takes on additional importance in health-related situations. Nonverbal messages flow continuously because of the human element. Words may not convey the total meaning of what a patient is trying to express. Whenever possible, the message should be validated. The nurse should make sure that the patient's communication has been understood. Mannerisms, expressions, and even odors convey a message. Patients who arrive on a unit dirty, disheveled, and unkempt tell us without speaking that they cannot care for themselves at an optimal level.

Generally speaking, if a sender and a receiver are willing to communicate, a message will be conveyed and shared. Sometimes patients ask questions that may be uncomfortable for nurses to answer. Sometimes nurses ask patients questions that the patients are unwilling to answer. When these situations occur, the nonverbal response in itself is a message. A basic premise of communication is that we cannot not communicate. Nonverbal responses, such as gestures or facial expressions, or the absence of gestures or facial expressions, may deliver a message.

For example, a woman whose terminal cancer has been diagnosed recently but who has not been told yet asks, "Nurse, am I dying?" The nurse, feeling unable to tell the patient the truth, does not respond at all. What do you think the patient feels? This nonverbal response may cause anxiety in the patient, because fear of the unknown is one of the greatest fears.

INTERPERSONAL SKILLS

Communicating well and appropriately both to get a point across and to understand another person requires good interpersonal skills. Interpersonal skills can be mastered by all who know and apply some general principles.

Therapeutic Tool

Psychiatric nursing skills are based on empathic listening, understanding the patient's internal frame of reference, and verbalizing emotional support and feedback, when appropriate. By applying these positive interpersonal skills in all their interactions with patients, nurses are using themselves as therapeutic tools. Just as cardiology nurses rely on electrocardiographic (ECG) machines for information, and surgical nurses apply sterile dressings to postoperative wounds to foster healing, so psychiatric nurses use their interpersonal and communication skills to continually assess patients and simultaneously provide therapeutic intervention to foster patients' emotional and mental health. General hospital staff nurses are in a position to easily tune into the emotional status of their patients.

The skills of listening, understanding, and verbalizing are not limited to psychiatric nurses. Like other skills, they can be learned by other specialty nurses. These skills allow nurses to respond more comfortably to the psychosocial as well as the physical needs of patients.

Considerations

Although the basic components needed for communication are simply a sender, a receiver, and a message, other factors also play a role in producing interactions that are accurate, successful, and positive.

Time. The time of day may make a difference for some interactions, particularly in the health field. Illnesses, accidents, and mishaps occur at all hours of the day and night. Additionally, hospitals, nursing homes, residential treatment facilities, and some home health situations are ongoing. Most nurses work within the framework of three shifts of 8 hr per shift or two shifts of 12 hr per 24 hr. At some time, every nurse probably has worked part, if not all, of a night shift.

The ambiance that exists on a medical-surgical unit during the day shift, when activity is plentiful—patients being seen by consultants, physicians, and therapists; taken for tests; and visited by friends and family—changes dramatically during the night. Often patients are more anxious during the night, because they have fewer distractions (both people and activities) from their concerns and fears. This anxiety could be one cause of a patient's sleeplessness or of the increase in requests for nursing attention. Nighttime may also be a good time for nurses to communicate with patients. Communication is no better or worse during the day or the night, but the differences between these two times should be considered.

Place. Where interactions occur also should be considered. Think about the environmental differences in the following health-related areas:

- Emergency department
- Operating room
- Nursing home
- Patient's private residence
- Doctor's office
- Pediatric clinic
- Ambulance
- Psychiatric unit

These are just some of the places nurses interact with patients. The needs of each patient and the pace of the health-related visit are different at each one. It follows that different places require different interpersonal skills for therapeutic interactions.

Person. Each human is unique. Although some of us have similarities, each of us is an individual.

Although some diseases and disorders are documented and diagnosed on the basis of the same signs and symptoms, each patient has unique feelings, thoughts, values, language, culture, attitudes, and personality. All these factors must be considered when nurses and patients interact. Using the same words and phrases over and over again with all patients in all situations may not always be therapeutic. For some, yes; but for others, no.

Consider the following two situations:

1. A 35-year-old woman with a severe abdominal pain is brought to the emergency department by her husband. She is crying and quite distraught. A nurse is able to take time to pat the woman's hand and say, "We're looking for what's wrong; we'll try to help you to feel better soon."

2. A 35-year-old man drives himself to the emergency department. He says that he is having severe stomach pains, and his demeanor is stoic. During his workup, he is visibly grimacing, and he begins shouting for people to hurry up. A nurse approaches him and says, "We're looking for what's wrong; we'll try to help you to feel better soon." The patient yells at the nurse, "Do something and shut up." He pushes the nurse aside, says that all of the staff are incompetent, and clearly is beginning to lose control.

Although comforting words were of help to the first patient, the same words were an irritant to the second patient. Consequently, nurses must assess each patient and situation individually and devise the appropriate communication strategy accordingly.

Situational variance. Although all patients who require health-related interactions may be anxious about their medical situation, different problems require different interpersonal techniques. Patients in critical situations generally want and need swift and efficient care. For these patients, short communications delivered with a comforting demeanor are best. Some patients may be out of touch with reality and misinterpret the words and actions of others. Interactions with these patients require special skills. A conscious awareness of choice of words is needed in these situations. When different factors for different people are considered within the framework of using positive interpersonal skills, therapeutic interaction and good communication are attainable.

STRATEGIES FOR EFFECTIVE COMMUNICATION

Effective communication and interpersonal skills take some work. In all health care related situations, nurses should be aware of their demeanor and verbal abilities as well as their limitations. Particularly in situations of psychiatric and psychosocial stress, nurses need to use these interpersonal skills to accomplish a therapeutic outcome.

Listening

Listening and the therapeutic use of silence are valuable tools. Active listening is achieved by paying close attention to the sender of the message. The listener should attend to the sender's verbal and nonverbal communication. Maintaining an attentive posture, changing facial expressions to conform with the content of what the patient is saying, using hand gestures, and nodding and shaking the head all convey attention. Some sounds have come to mean specific things:

- Ah hah!
- Uh oh!
- Uh huh?

These commonly used phrases encourage interactions.

Silence is therapeutic when it is used to convey an interest in what the patient is saying. Listening without interrupting tells the patient that you want to hear more.

Feedback and Clarification

At some time, everyone has spoken at length about something only to hear from the listener a question or statement that is completely off target. Clarifying what is being said, heard, and understood by both parties should be ongoing in communication. This clarification is achieved by giving and receiving feedback.

Clear communication can be achieved by doing the following:

- Asking questions
- Answering questions
- Summarizing what you have heard
- Probing for more information if needed
- Giving more information as requested

Reflection can also be used to confirm what has been said. With this technique, the listener repeats in a questioning manner part of what has been said. Consider the following examples:

- You said that hurt?
- You could not hear?
- You're feeling nervous?

Reflection is a commonly used tool that successfully encourages patients to continue with what they were saying.

Questioning Techniques

Nurses continually need information from patients. Sometimes direct questions are appropriate. Consider the following examples:

- Are you in pain?
- Did you sleep last night?

In some situations, more often in the psychiatric realm, it is desirable to hear in detail what a patient is feeling and thinking. At these times, open-ended questions are helpful. Open-ended questions are phrased in such a way that they cannot be answered with a simple yes or no; they require some added content. Consider the following examples:

- And then?
- What do you mean by that?
- What happened next?
- Can you tell me more about it?
- When? Where? How?

Support and Reassurance

Care and nurturance are integral aspects of nursing. Providing support and realistic reassurance to patients at times of crisis for the patients is a valuable intervention.

Support and reassurance can be given through the use of comforting words, gestures, and facial expressions. A discriminating use of touch, such as a pat on the hand or a slight touch on the shoulder, and being at the patient's side are helpful. Essentially, you want to convey to patients that you understand them and are concerned for them and interested in them, without offering false hope and promises. Knowledge about their situation and mastery of their own behavior helps patients achieve a sense of well-being even while hospitalized.

Table 1-1 gives some phrases that are helpful for open communication. *Table 1-2* gives some that tend to close communication. Each nurse should use statements, phrases, questions, and gestures that are comfortable and natural for him or her.

BARRIERS TO COMMUNICATION

Several problems in interaction and communication may arise when nurses are with patients.

Foreign Language

In the United States, many people speak foreign languages. Some immigrated a long time ago but have never learned English. Some may understand English but not speak it well. Everyday, non–English-speaking people come to this country to live, work, or visit. Some states share borders with Mexico and Canada, where people speak Spanish or French as well as English. Sometimes, elderly persons who have spoken English as a second language revert to their native tongue. This reversion also may happen when someone is highly stressed, in great pain, delirious, possibly demented, or psychotic.

How many times have you shouted at a patient who does not speak English? Obviously shouting is not helpful, and often it eliminates the patient's interest in trying to communicate. These patients will not understand you better because you are louder; after all, they are not hard of hearing. They may be offended by your shouting, and communication may be blocked even more.

Possible alternatives include the following:

- Use an interpreter, preferably one with a medical background. Some institutions maintain a list of employees who speak foreign languages.

- Ask a relative or friend of the patient to interpret. In some situations, it is necessary to know the relationship between the patient and the interpreter, because the patient may be unwilling to be truthful with the interpreter. Usually a family member is the best choice.

- Use facial and hand gestures as well as good body language.

- Use pictures and graphs. Paper and chalkboards can be used for pointing to and drawing.

In a region that has many non–English-speaking patients, it is beneficial to learn the foreign language or a wide range of the vocabulary used in patients' care. A pocket-size translation book can

---

Table 1-1
Helpful Phrases for Open Communication

Support and Reassurance
Good job! Nice work!
I understand.
You seem better to me today. How are you?
How frustrating for you.
What a difficult situation this is.

Feedback and Clarification
I don't understand.
I don't know what you mean by that.
I am not following your train of thought.
Did you mean _____?
What about that…?
I cannot answer that question, I am not comfortable answering you, or I'd rather not answer that.

Exploring, Questioning, Probing, and Interpreting
What are you feeling?
What are you thinking about?
You seem to be seeing things or hearing voices. Are you?
You seem angry.
It appears to me as though you have been _____.
Have you been thinking about hurting yourself?
Go on.
And then?
Tell me more about that!

---

be an aid.

Generally, communicating with someone who speaks in another language is difficult but not totally useless for obtaining some data for initial assessment and for providing support. It is better to make an attempt so the patient does not feel isolated, ignored, or anxious.

Ethnic and Cultural Issues

Like those with language barriers, persons with different ethnic backgrounds and other cultural influences require special attention. Even though they may speak English, the interpretation of language and the meanings ascribed to symbols, attitudes, and facial expressions associated with different medical issues and procedures may seem different from what is familiar to us. It is easy for nurses to misinterpret persons from different cultures, a situation than ensures some negative interactions.

Persons from different backgrounds may respond to pain differently. Some are stoic; others need to "let out" their emotions.

Some cultures aspire to maintain dignity by not exerting independence. For others, the opposite is true, and maintaining distance from others is more the rule.

Some cultures use symbols, medicinal herbs and potions, and trinkets. Although they may seem trivial to the nurse, these may be extremely important to a patient's sense of well-being.

Some persons have tremendous faith in their religion and request a visit from a member of their church. Others may have a belief in spiritual healing and cures and make use of ceremonial acts, rites, or visits.

Understanding that a basic difference does exist, avoiding "jumping to conclusions" about the patient, and attempting to understand the cultural issues will help produce successful interactions. You may want to try the following:

- Talk openly with patients. Ask them to explain what you think of as "strange" behavior. Be nonjudgmental, observational, curious.

- Ask others such as visitors or coworkers who may be of the same faith, culture, or background as the patient about things that may confuse you.

- Become more knowledgeable; read about other cultures.

- Be open to others' points of view. It is not necessary to agree with them; just try to see things

Table 1-2
Phrases That Close Communication

False Promises
I'll be back in a few minutes (not returning).

Rejecting and Disapproving
That's wrong.
Don't tell me that.
I don't believe you.
You can't be right.
It must be this way.

Challenging
You can't be seeing pink elephants.
There are no loud voices. You can't be hearing them.
If the FBI is after you, why haven't they caught you yet?
You don't look like God.

Defensiveness
How can you say that? Why, this is the finest hospital!

Discounting the Patient's Feelings
You can't be upset about that?
Everyone feels blue sometimes.

from their perspective and be empathic.

- When interacting, ask for feedback and clarification. Find out whether you understand correctly and whether you are being understood correctly. Ask the patient to repeat what you have said, and repeat what the patient says to you.

- Be flexible. Perhaps some hospital routines can be changed or modified for the patient's benefit. This in turn helps the nurse.

Like people who speak a foreign language, people of different cultural backgrounds may feel quite isolated in an unfamiliar environment. The nurse who is at the patient's bedside for a substantial time can be helpful by using interpersonal skills therapeutically.

Mutism

Some patients pose a special problem because they do not speak, or they speak little and seldom. Some patients are mute and cannot speak because of a physical disorder or disability. Some psychiatric disturbances leave patients incapable of speech or unwilling to talk.

It is important to discern why a patient is not speaking. The reason may be included in the patient's records, known by the patient's friends or relatives, or conveyed by the patient in sign language. If a patient cannot speak, nonverbal gestures and written communications can be used. When a patient is unwilling to communicate, the nurse must consider why. Is the patient fearful and afraid; psychotic and not in touch with reality; desperately sad and depressed; or perhaps angry, hostile, and negative?

The following approaches may be useful:

- Make time to be with the patient. Try not to be rushed or too pushy.

- Set a time in advance to meet with the patient: "I'll be back in 15 minutes to sit with you. Perhaps you will share some of your concerns with me then?" This approach allows the patient to prepare for the interview. If you are not successful the first time, try again later.

- Sit quietly with the patient: "I'll just sit here with you and keep you company for a few minutes. We don't need to talk." This approach tells the patient you are willing to be with him or her without the pressure of speaking.

- Determine the appropriate amount of time to spend with the patient. Short, frequent contacts (i.e., 5 min every 30–60 min) may be most comfortable for the patient and the nurse.

- Be supportive but not overbearing. Allow for some of the distancing needs the patient may have.

Interaction with a mute patient is obviously difficult. However, once the cause of the mutism is determined, some form of communication will succeed.

Pain

Patients who are in mild, moderate, or severe pain may have difficulty maintaining interactions in a normal manner. The entire focus of attention of people in pain is generally themselves, their pain, and ways to seek relief from pain. This preoccupation may create a barrier to the flow of communication. In this situation, nurses bear the burden of maintaining the interaction, of being flexible and being able to forego interaction when necessary. They should be alert for cues that indicate the patient is willing and able to communicate and then communicate at those times.

Lethargy

Patients who are lethargic do not communicate as accurately and astutely as they normally do. Ways to overcome this barrier include the following:

- Assess the patient's level of consciousness.

- Ask the patient first if this is a good time to talk; then assess the patient's ability to maintain a conversation.

- Get feedback about the patient's understanding of what you are discussing.

- If the patient is too lethargic, wait for another time. The patient may be unable to sustain the interaction.

Anxiety

Many patients who are in a general hospital experience anxiety on one level or another. Communicating with anxious patients requires some special attention. Someone who is highly anxious may not be able to pay enough attention to hear and interpret language correctly. Because anxiety is so common, and because nurses are in a key posi-

tion to help patients cope with and alleviate some of it and its sequelae, it is reviewed in chapter 3.

Confusion

Confusion presents a severe barrier to accurate communication. Chapter 8 discusses the appropriate nursing interventions for patients who are confused.

Psychosis

Patients who are psychotic (i.e., out of touch with reality and perhaps delusional or hallucinating) cannot judge interactions appropriately. Chapter 6 has more information on the nursing management of patients who are psychotic.

SUMMARY

Generally speaking, nurses who genuinely care about patients and who use some basic knowledge about effective interpersonal skills manage to communicate quite appropriately with psychiatric patients. Nonpsychiatric nurses often are afraid they may say the wrong thing and thereby harm the patient or put words into the patient's mouth or thoughts into the patient's head. This is usually not the case. The techniques covered in this chapter are useful with all patients regardless of the patients' diagnosis.

EXAM QUESTIONS

CHAPTER 1
Questions 1–8

1. The process of communication is best characterized as:

   a. Stationary

   b. Multidimensional

   c. Motivational

   d. Ongoing

2. What are the three basic components needed for communication?

   a. Sender, listener, receiver

   b. Receiver, message, feedback

   c. Sender, receiver, message

   d. Feedback, listener, message

3. Which of the following is a basic premise in communication?

   a. The sender of a message is a nurse.

   b. We use body language.

   c. We cannot NOT communicate.

   d. Feedback occurs.

4. The patient is a youth with a large extended family who live nearby. The family visit much of the day and refuse to leave the unit when asked. The rules of the hospital specify visiting hours; the patient clearly seems better when his family is around. Which of the following is an appropriate nursing intervention?

   a. Get permission to extend the visiting hours for the family.

   b. Request help from the security staff.

   c. Be firm and assertive; tell the family to leave

   d. Turn your back; make believe the family members are not there.

5. Which of the following is a psychiatric nurse's best therapeutic tool?

   a. Sphygmomanometer

   b. Good language skills

   c. Method of observation

   d. Herself or himself

6. How is active listening achieved?

   a. By using hand gestures

   b. By getting feedback

   c. By saying Oh no!

   d. By paying close attention

7. Which of the following is <u>not a</u> helpful phrase for open communication?

     a. I understand.

     b. No!

     c. I don't understand

     d. And then?

8. Which of the following is an example of a phrase that will close communication?

     a. I understand.

     b. Did you mean _____?

     c. Tell me more about that!

     d. You can't be upset by that!

CHAPTER 2

HOW TO ASSESS PSYCHOSOCIAL PROBLEMS

CHAPTER OBJECTIVE

After completing this chapter, the reader will be able to differentiate assessment tools and specify their components.

LEARNING OBJECTIVES

After studying this chapter, the reader will be able to

1. Specify one reason assessment of patients is important.

2. Recognize major components of a mental status examination.

3. Specify components of a mini–mental status examination.

4. Indicate the major components of a psychosocial assessment.

5. Specify the four major components of the nursing process used as a standard in psychiatric nursing.

6. Recognize the major psychosocial nursing diagnoses.

7. Recognize DSM-IV diagnoses.

ASSESSMENT

Assessment of patients with psychiatric and psychosocial problems is a critical step in the nursing process. Sometimes nurses work with patients who are highly stressed, confused in thinking, or behaving in an uncontrolled, irrational manner. These situations call for skill in interpersonal communications.

Assessments are used to determine patients' problems, get to know patients and their coping skills, and plan nursing interventions. Each institution or agency generally specifies which assessment tool is used. It is standard procedure to thoroughly assess each patient when the patient first enters a nursing unit. If you are not the admitting nurse, it is incumbent on you to review the admission intake summary provided by your colleague.

Assessing patients is an ongoing process. Although an entire assessment form need not be completed each shift, day, or week, observing changes in patients during each shift is part of the assessment process.

Observation skills include using some of the senses:

• Hearing: What is the patient saying or not saying? Are there any strange noises?

• Sense of smell: Are any odors emanating from the patient or the patient's belongings or the room?

• Sense of touch: Touching patients is more common when they have physical problems, which may require hands-on care such as dressing changes and physical rather than psychiatric monitoring. However, many patients have more than one problem.

Both the patient and the patient's immediate environment should be observed. Patients' belongings may tell us something about them or the people who are with them or, if a patient is alone, give us some social information. In all cases, we learn something.

In home care situations, a thorough assessment of the patient's environment is critical. Specific safety factors should be checked. Patients' general life-style and ability to care for themselves at home are ongoing considerations. An important consideration is their ability to manage their own medications. A great deal of information about a patient's personal life, culture, likes, and dislikes can be gleaned in the home. When assessment takes place in an outpatient setting, private office, or clinic, factors such as hygiene, grooming, and ability to travel to and from appointments are additional considerations.

All observations are valuable. Some are especially important. Others are less crucial. The best strategy is to gather all the information available and prioritize it later when planning care.

MENTAL STATUS EXAMINATION

The mental status examination *(Table 2-1)* is the part of the clinical assessment that describes the sum total of the examiner's observations and impressions of the psychiatric patient at the time of the interview (Kaplan & Sadock, 1991). This examination is used by many members of the various health care disciplines as the foundation for assessing a psychiatric patient. Different formats are used. Some are quite detailed; others, such as mini mental status examinations, are more abbreviated. Nurses who work in an agency that uses a standardized format through-

out its various departments should use the format that is most familiar to them. When all the information is gathered, a fairly extensive description of the patient's current emotional state and thought processes will be available.

MINI–MENTAL STATUS EXAMINATION

A mini–mental status examination can range from finding out if the patient is oriented to time, place, and person to a more detailed format such as the Cognitive Capacity Screening Examination *(Table 2-2)*.

CASE STUDY

The following vignette describes a patient and presents the mental status examination as it might be written on a chart *(Table 2-3)*.

You are the day nurse on a medical unit. A woman was admitted to your unit last evening from the emergency department. Her diagnosis is pneumonia. She has begun taking antibiotics and makes no complaints. You notice that she is crying, and she denies being in any pain. You feel that something is not right with this patient, and you make some time to do a mental status examination.

While talking with the patient, you acquire additional information that is necessary for a more complete assessment: The patient says she has been sleeping a lot, has a small appetite, and cannot remember when she has been hungry for a full meal. The chart reveals a history of early morning awakening; this is corroborated by the night nursing notes, which report that the patient awakened at 3:10 a.m. Her record states she has lost 5 lb (2.3 kg) in the past month. She says she lives alone; her husband died 9 months ago. She has one son who lives 35 miles away and a daughter in another state. She speaks with them on the telephone but does not get to see them much. She has some friends but

Table 2-1
Components of the Mental Status Examination

General Appearance
Description of the patient's physical characteristics
    Apparent age
    Grooming
        Hygiene (e.g., clean, dirty, disheveled)
        Dress (e.g., neat, careless, bizarre)
        Posture

Behavior and Psychomotor Status
Patient's body language, movements, and facial expressions
    Stereotyped behavior
    Gait
    Gestures
    Mannerisms
    Movements: Types and speed (e.g., agitated, restless), tremors, coarse or fine psychomotor retardation, wringing of hands

Attitude Toward Interviewer
Patient's attitude (e.g., attentive, friendly or angry, dramatic or muted, cooperative, suspicious, hostile, passive, dependent, indifferent, seductive)

Affect and Mood
Description of the patient's emotional state
    Affect: the patient's expression of his or her emotional state (e.g., facial expression)
    Words used to describe affect include blunted, flat, normal range, constricted.
    Mood: The pervasive and sustained emotion of the person
    Words used to describe mood include sad, angry, happy, depressed, worried, nervous, suspicious, dull, hostile, elated, apathetic.

Speech
Characteristics of how the patient talks
    Quantity
    Rate of production
    Quality
Words used to describe speech include pressured, rapid, talkative, lacking spontaneity.

Thought Content/Perceptual Disturbances
Assessments for disturbed thought processes or perceptual disturbances, or difficulty and strangeness in thinking, especially for two major problems: delusions and hallucinations.

    Delusion: A fixed, false belief. For example, "The Mafia is out to get me", or "I am Jesus Christ."
    Hallucination: False sensory data. Hallucinations can be visual, auditory, olfactory, gustatory, or tactile. The most common types are hearing voices or seeing visions or both.

Sensorium and Cognition
Orientation of the patient to time, place, and person: Essentially, we are asking if the patient knows who he or she is, where he or she is, and when this time is.
Alertness and level of consciousness: Does the patient's sensorium seem clear, or is it clouded and confused?
Memory: Assessment of three time frames
    Immediate: Can be tested by asking the patient to remember three items for a few minutes; for example, "I am going to ask you to remember a key, a book, and a lamp; I'll ask you again later." Move on with other questions and then say, "This is a good time to try and remember the three objects I mentioned before."
    Recent: Can the patient tell you, with considerable detail and accuracy, the events that led up to the hospitalization?
    Remote: Refers to the patient's distant personal history. This type of memory is the most difficult to check for accuracy. Some simple questions may be ones about the patient's upbringing, where he or she lived, where he or she went to school.

General Fund of Knowledge
General information such as the name of the president of the United States, the name of the governor of the state where the patient lives, answers to simple mathematical calculations.

Insight and Judgment
Can be checked for by listening (1) to the patient describe what he or she thinks is happening to him or her at the present time and how he or she perceives his or her illness and (2) to what decisions the patient is making with regard to the current situation.

Source: Kaplan, H. I., & Sadock, B. J. (1991). Synopsis of psychiatry: *Behavioral sciences clinical psychiatry* (6th ed.). Baltimore: Williams & Wilkins.

Table 2-2
Cognitive Capacity Screening Examination

Examiner _____
Date _____

Addressograph Plate

Instructions: Check items answered correctly. Write incorrect or unusual answers in space provided. If necessary, urge patient once to complete task.

Introduction to patient: "I would like to ask you a few questions. Some you will find very easy and others may be very hard. Just do your best."

1) What day of the week is this? _____
2) What month? _____
3) What day of month? _____
4) What year? _____
5) What place is this? _____
6) Repeat the numbers 8 7 2. _____
7) Say them backwards. _____
8) Repeat these numbers 6 8 7 1. _____
9) Listen to these numbers 6 9 4. Count 1 through 10 out loud, then repeat 6 9 4. (Help if needed. Then use numbers 5 7 3.) _____
10) Listen to these numbers 8 1 4 3. Count 1 through 10 out loud, then repeat 8 1 4 3. _____
11) Beginning with Sunday, say the days of the week backwards. _____
12) 9 + 3 is _____
13) Add 6 (to the previous answer or "to 12"). _____
14) Take away 5 ("from 18"). _____
Repeat these words after me and remember them. I will ask for them later: HAT, CAR, TREE, TWENTY-SIX. _____

15) The opposite of fast is slow. The opposite of up is _____
16) The opposite of large is _____
17) The opposite of hard is _____
18) An orange and a banana are both fruits. Red and blue are both _____
19) A penny and a dime are both _____
20) What were those words I asked you to remember? (HAT). _____
21) (CAR) _____
22) (TREE) _____
23) (TWENTY-SIX) _____
24) Take away 7 from 100, then take away 7 from what is left and keep going: 100-7 is _____
25) Minus 7 _____
26) Minus 7 (write down answers; check correct subtraction of 7) _____
27) Minus 7 _____
28) Minus 7 _____
29) Minus 7 _____
30) Minus 7 _____
TOTAL CORRECT (maximum score =30) _____

Patient's occupation (previous if not employed) _____ Education _____ Age _____
Estimated intelligence (based on eduation, occupation, and history, not on test score): Below average, Average, Above average _____
Patient was: Cooperative ___ Uncooperative ___ Depressed ___ Lethargic ___ Other _____
Medical Diagnosis: _____

IF PATIENT'S SCORE IS LESS THAN 20, THE EXISTENCE OF DIMINISHED COGNITIVE CAPACITY IS PRESENT. THEREFORE, AN ORGANIC MENTAL SYNDROME SHOULD BE SUSPECTED AND THE FOLLOWING INFORMATION OBTAINED.

Temp. _____   BUN _____
B.P. _____   Glu _____
Hct _____   Po2 _____
Na _____   Pco2 _____
K _____
Cl _____
CO2 _____
EEG _____
ECG _____

Endocrine dysfunction? _____
T3, T4, Ca, P, etc.

History of previous psychiatric difficulty _____

Drugs: _____
Steroids? L-Dopa? Amphetamines? Tranquilizers? Digitalis?

Focal neurological signs: _____

DIAGNOSIS: _____

·From: Screening for Organic Metal Syndrome in the Medically Ill. by J. W. Jacobs, M. R. Bernhard, A. Delgado, and J. J. Strain, *Annals of Internal Medicine*, 1977. Reprinted with permission.

mental status examination, you accurately decide that this patient has a mood disorder, with signs and symptoms of depression. The nursing diagnoses include one or more of the following:

- Self-esteem disturbance
- Social isolation
- Powerlessness
- Altered nutrition, less than body requirements
- Sleep pattern disturbance
- Diversional activity deficit
- Adjustment, impaired
- Individual coping, ineffective
- Self-care deficit: bathing/hygiene

PSYCHOSOCIAL ASSESSMENT

The mental status examination is only one part of a complete psychosocial assessment. The complete assessment includes a history-taking procedure and a nursing assessment that reviews the patient's past, present, and future goals, encompassing physical, psychological, and social components *(Table 2-4)*. The psychosocial assessment is the foundation for the nursing process, and although a great deal of information is included immediately, additional information can be obtained later on. Many agencies use a standardized format, and this may be part of a nursing care plan or part of a patient's complete record.

generally feels too tired to see them. She claims she is not a joiner, and she does not participate in any community activities or church groups. She has always been a housewife, never working outside her home, and says, "I don't imagine I could do much of anything else."

On the basis of all of the data collected and the

NURSING STRATEGIES FOR ASSESSING PSYCHOSOCIAL PROBLEMS

Setting a Time Frame

It seems obvious that obtaining a thorough psychosocial assessment can be a lengthy process, and in nursing, time is precious. Therefore, a time frame should be chosen accordingly. Although an initial assessment done when the patient arrives is useful immediately, all the information required need not be obtained then. Some basic information can be obtained when the patient arrives, and the rest can be acquired later in a more relaxed manner. A rushed interview is doomed to failure, both in gathering information and in using the opportunity to begin establishing a rapport with the patient.

Ensuring Confidentiality

The most appropriate place for interviewing a patient is in private, so attempt to obtain the psychosocial history with as few people present as possible. If you are in a semiprivate room, close all curtains or dividers. Perhaps the patient is ambulatory or perhaps the patient's roommate might leave. There may be much information that a patient will be uncomfortable talking about in the presence of others, even family members or friends.

Patients deserve the right to confidentiality in what they tell you. You should reassure them about confidentiality at the beginning of the interview. You should be careful not to divulge any information in an unethical manner. Patients should not be discussed with anyone who is not a participant in their treatment.

Documenting Findings

The nursing psychosocial assessment should be included in the patient's permanent record of care. This information will be shared with other members of the multidisciplinary health team.

Establishing Therapeutic Relationships

The initial intake period offers ample opportunity to begin a therapeutic relationship with the patient. Show sensitivity and respect while communicating with patients. An empathic demeanor will indicate caring and interest.

An awareness of your own insecurities or anxieties about the patient should also be considered. Be alert to any potentially dangerous behaviors for the sake of the patient's safety as well as your own. If you are calm, patient, and interested, assessment can provide the foundation for therapeutic nursing care.

THE NURSING PROCESS

Psychiatric nursing, although a specialty with its own standards of care as specified by the American Nurses' Association, uses a process consisting of systematic steps toward the delivery of care that are based on the science and art of nursing theory and practice. The process has four components:

1. **Assessment:** Gathering and analyzing verbal and nonverbal information through history taking and observation

2. **Plan:** Establishing goals with the patient and developing strategies for achieving them

3. **Implementation:** Using nursing interventions to attain goals

4. **Evaluation:** Critically reviewing goal achievement: total, partial, or none

The nursing process is an integral part of psychiatric nursing and of the delivery of psychosocial nursing care to all patients.

Table 2-3
Example of a Mental Status Examination

Interviewer: M. Nadler-Moodie, R.N. **Date:** _____

General Appearance: Elderly white woman, appearing her stated age of 69 years old, is dressed in a hospital gown, socks, and a bed jacket. Hair is gray and unkempt, she wears no makeup, her fingernails are long and dirty with some food particles.

Motor Status and Affect: When she is ambulating to the bathroom, the patient's gait is slow and unsteady. She is slightly tremulous and holds onto the wall for support. Her posture is stooped. Facies appear sad. She has poor eye contact, little or no smiling. Affect is blunted with low range, no spontaneity.

General Behavior: Patient lies quietly in bed, either sleeping or with her eyes closed. She's been wringing her hands.

Speech and Language: Speech is very soft and slow; she answers questions in monosyllables. No incoherence noted or any illogical or strange words elicited. Native language is English.

Mood: Often teary-eyed and appears to be depressed. When asked about her mood, she replies, "I'm just very tired, and I do feel a bit down."

Thought Content: Some difficulty concentrating. Denies any special thoughts, delusions, or hallucinations. Denies any suicidal ideation, but is morbid in her thinking, saying, "I'm old and sick, and I suppose I won't live very much longer."

Orientation: Oriented x 3: Correct on person and place, slightly off on date, thinking today is "9-24-89."

Memory: Recent memory fair to good. Can recall events leading to hospitalization. Remote: good recall of past history.

General Fund of Knowledge: Completed high school, gives information correctly, seems of average intelligence. Accurate on simple calculations; thinks abstractly to people in glass houses…responds, "You shouldn't criticize someone for doing something you do as well."

Insight: Insight seems poor: doesn't seem to understand the nature of depression as possible contribution to her declining health.

Additional Comments:

NURSING DIAGNOSES

As part of a complete psychosocial nursing assessment, nursing diagnoses have been used increasingly as one means of standardizing nursing practice. Nurses who are committed to achieving this standardization have established the North American Nursing Diagnosis Association (NANDA). NANDA publishes an updated list of nursing diagnoses on a biannual basis. The current list (1995–1996) has 129 entries *(Table 2-5)*. The association continues to work on researching and developing new and refined nursing diagnoses as research directs.

DIAGNOSTIC AND STATISTICAL MANUAL OF MENTAL DISORDERS

The psychiatric diagnoses that are specified solely or along with medical diagnoses as part of a patient's permanent medical record are based on the *Diagnostic and Statistical Manual of Mental Disorders* (DSM-IV; American Psychiatric Association, 1994). The diagnostic groupings most likely to be seen in general hospital nursing are as follows:

* Delirium, dementia, and other cognitive disorders

* Substance-related disorders

* Mood disorders

* Psychotic disorders

* Anxiety disorders

* Somatoform disorders

* Adjustment disorders

* Mental disorders due to a general medical condition

* Personality disorders

* Eating disorders

The appendix contains a complete list of the DSM-IV diagnoses and codes.

Table 2-4
Components of a Psychosocial Assessment

General Information
Includes demographic information and identifying data.
Name
Address
Date of birth
Sex
Race, ethnic background, cultural beliefs
Religion, background, beliefs, practices
Marital status

Presenting Problem
What is the patient's chief complaint? This generally is stated in the patient's own words, and should be quotable.

History of Problem
When did it begin?
What is the nature of the problem (e.g., signs and symptoms, concerns)?
Any events or occurrences that may have led to the problem?
Present therapeutic contacts (i.e., therapy with physician, nurse, psychologist, social worker, other).

Has this problem occurred before?
Pertinent personal psychiatric history?
Pertinent family history?
Relevant past counseling?

Medical History
Past or present medical problems?
Pertinent family history?
Physician or other health-related visits?
Laboratory values: Any known, recent work on chart, other?

Socioeconomic Background
Family system
Occupation Education level: What was last completed school grade?
Financial, including information on health insurance
Habits: Eating, drinking, smoking, drug use, personal hygiene

Sexual History
General activity
Preference

Table 2.4 *(Continued)*

Support Systems	**Possible Normal Responses**
Friends	Talk with someone.
Family	Ignore it.
Affiliations	Withdraw.
Leisure time activity	Get angry and yell.
	Get angry and be quiet.
Level of Stress During the Year Before Admission	Get angry and hit/throw something.
Changes in work or school (e.g., promotion, demotion, firing, graduation, change of job or school)?	Drink.
	Become anxious.
	Become depressed.
Change in the family (e.g., death, divorce, birth of new·baby, child leaving home, change in residence, change in financial status)?	**Developmental History:**
	Include any pertinent childhood adolescent issues
Normal Coping Ability	*Medications*
How does the patient normally cope?	Currently taking?
What conscious coping strategies does the patient use when severely stressed?	Past responses and reactions
Possible Questions:	Known allergies
"When you experience stress in your everyday life, what do you do to decrease it?"	Over-the-counter medications frequently taken
"When you go through a very rough time, how do you normally handle it?"	*Significant Events*
	Any other occurrences, losses not yet mentioned?

Table 2-5

North American Nursing Diagnoses Association 1995–1996 List of Nursing Diagnoses

Pattern 1:	Exchanging
1.1.2.1	Altered nutrition: more than body requirements
1.1.2.2	Altered nutrition: less than body requirements
1.1.2.3	Altered nutrition: potential for more than body requirements
1.2.1.1	Risk for Infection
1.2.2.1	Risk for altered body temperature
1.2.2.2	Hypothermia
1.2.2.3	Hyperthermia
1.2.2.4	Ineffective thermoregulation
1.2.3.1	Dysreflexia
1.3.1.1	Constipation
1.3.1.1.1	Perceived constipation
1.3.1.1.2	Colonic constipation
1.3.1.2	Diarrhea
1.3.1.3	Bowel incontinence
1.3.2	Altered urinary elimination
1.3.2.1.1	Stress incontinence
1.3.2.1.2	Reflex incontinence
1.3.2.1.3	Urge incontinence
1.3.2.1.3	Functional incontinence
1.3.2.1.5	Total incontinence
1.3.2.2	Urinary retention
1.4.1.1	Altered (specify type) tissue perfusion (renal, cerebral, cardiopulmonary, gastrointestinal, peripheral)
1.4.1.2.1	Fluid volume excess
1.4.1.2.2.1	Fluid volume deficit
1.4.1.2.2.2	Risk for fluid volume deficit
1.4.2.1	Decreased cardiac output
1.5.1.1	Impaired gas exchange
1.5.1.2	Ineffective airway clearance
1.5.1.3	Ineffective breathing pattern
1.5.1.3.1	Inability to sustain spontaneous ventilation
1.5.1.3.2	Dysfunctional ventilatory weaning response (DVWR)
1.6.1	Risk for injury
1.6.1.1	Risk for suffocation
1.6.1.2	Risk for poisoning
1.6.1.3	Risk for trauma
1.6.1.4	Risk for aspiration
1.6.1.5	Risk for disuse syndrome
1.6.2	Altered protection
1.6.2.1	Impaired tissue integrity
1.6.2.1.1	Altered oral mucous membrane
1.6.2.1.2.1	Impaired skin injury
1.6.2.1.2.2	Risk for impaired skin integrity

Table 2-5 *(Continued)*

1.7.1	Decreased adaptive capacity: intracranial
1.8	Energy field disturbance

Pattern 2: Communicating

2.1.1.1	Impaired verbal communication

Pattern 3: Relating

3.1.1	Impaired social interaction
3.1.2	Social isolation
3.1.3	Risk for loneliness
3.2.1	Altered role performance
3.2.1.1.1	Altered parenting
3.2.1.1.2.1	Risk for altered parent/infant/child attachment
3.2.1.2.1	Sexual dysfunction
3.2.2	Altered family processes
3.2.2.1	Caregiver role strain
3.2.2.2	Risk for caregiver role strain
3.2.2.3.1	Altered family process: alcoholism
3.2.3.1	Parental role conflict
3.3	Altered sexual patterns

Pattern 4: Valuing

4.1.1	Spiritual distress (distress of the human spirit)
4.2	Potential for enhanced spiritual well-being

Pattern 5: Choosing

5.1.1.1	Ineffective individual coping
5.1.1.1.1	Impaired adjustment
5.1.1.1.2	Defensive coping
5.1.1.1.3	Ineffective denial
5.1.2.1.1	Ineffective family coping: disabling
5.1.2.1.2	Ineffective family coping: compromised
5.1.2.2	Family coping: potential for growth
5.1.3.1	Potential for enhanced community coping
5.1.3.2	Ineffective community coping
5.2.1	Ineffective management of therapeutic regimen (individuals)
5.2.1.1	Noncompliance (specify)
5.2.2	Ineffective management of therapeutic regimen: families
5.2.3	Ineffective management of therapeutic regimen: community
5.2.4	Ineffective management of therapeutic regimen: individual
5.3.1.1	Decisional conflict (specify)
5.4	Health-seeking behaviors (specify)

Table 2-5 *(Continued)*

Pattern 6:	**Moving**
6.1.1.1	Impaired physical mobility
6.1.1.1.1	Risk for peripheral neurovascular dysfunction
6.1.1.1.2	Risk for perioperative positioning injury
6.1.1.2	Activity intolerance
6.1.1.2.1	Fatigue
6.1.1.3	Risk for activity intolerance
6.2.1	Sleep pattern disturbance
6.3.1.1	Diversional activity deficit
6.4.1.1	Impaired home maintenance management
6.4.2	Altered health maintenance
6.5.1	Feeding self-care deficit
6.5.1.1	Impaired swallowing
6.5.1.2	Ineffective breastfeeding
6.5.1.2.1	Interrupted breastfeeding
6.5.1.3	Effective breastfeeding
6.5.1.4	Ineffective infant feeding pattern
6.5.2	Bathing/hygiene self-care deficit
6.5.3	Dressing/grooming self-care deficit
6.5.4	Toileting self-care deficit
6.6	Altered growth and development
6.7	Relocation stress syndrome
6.8.1	Risk for disorganized infant behavior
6.8.2	Disorganized infant behavior
6.8.3	Potential for enhanced organized infant behavior
Pattern 7:	**Perceiving**
7.1.1	Body image disturbance
7.1.2	Self-esteem disturbance
7.1.2.1	Chronic low self-esteem
7.1.2.2	Situational low self-esteem
7.1.3	Personal identity disturbance
7.2	Sensory/perceptual alterations (specify) (visual, auditory, kinesthetic, gustatory, tactile, olfactory)
7.2.1.1	Unilateral neglect
7.3.1	Hopelessness
7.3.2	Powerlessness
Pattern 8:	**Knowing**
8.1.1	Knowledge deficit (specify)
8.2.1	Impaired environmental interpretation syndrome
8.2.2	Acute confusion
8.2.3	Chronic confusion
8.3	Altered thought processes
8.3.1	Impaired memory

Table 2-5 *(Continued)*

Pattern 9:	**Feeling**
9.1.1	Pain
9.1.1.1	Chronic Pain
9.2.1.1	Dysfunctional grieving
9.2.1.2	Anticipatory grieving
9.2.2	Risk for violence: Self-directed or directed at others
9.2.2.1	Risk for self-mutilation
9.2.3	Post-trauma response
9.2.3.1	Rape-trauma syndrome
9.2.3.1.1	Rape-trauma syndrome: compound reaction
9.2.3.1.2	Rape-trauma syndrome: silent reaction
9.3.1	Anxiety
9.3.2	Fear

EXAM QUESTIONS

CHAPTER 2

Questions 9–15

9. Assessing a patient is important because it allows the nurse to do which of the following?

    a. Report and document.

    b. Provide support and reassurance.

    c. Complete charting requirements.

    d. Determine the patient's problem and plan interventions.

10. Which of the following is an example of a mini–mental status examination?

    a. Cognitive Capacity Screening Examination

    b. Asking if the patient is oriented to time

    c. Psychological history

    d. DSM-IV

11. A psychosocial assessment includes which of the following?

    a. Medical history, treatment plan, confidentiality

    b. Language, orientation, sexual history

    c. Significant events, sexual history, motor status

    d. General information, medical history, socioeconomic background

12. An example of a nursing strategy for assessing a psychosocial problem would be for the nurse to do which of the following?

    a. Complete a nursing assessment.

    b. Maintain good eye contact.

    c. Establish a therapeutic relationship.

    d. Do a mental status examination.

13. NANDA is the acronym for which of the following?

    a. North American Nursing Diagnosis Association

    b. National Action for Nursing Diagnosis in America

    c. National Association for Nursing Diagnosis in America

    d. North American National Diagnostic Action

14. Which of the following is *not* a psychosocial nursing diagnosis?

    a. Fear

    b. Energy field disturbance

    c. Obsessive-compulsive disorder

    d. Anxiety

15. What are the four basic components of the nursing process?

  a. Assessment, plan, implementation, evaluation

  b. Observation, plan, implementation, evaluation

  c. Communication, message, receiver, sender

  d. Plan, interventions, observation, assessment

CHAPTER 3

NURSING MANAGEMENT OF THE ANXIOUS PATIENT

CHAPTER OBJECTIVE

After completing this chapter, the reader will be able to indicate how the concept of anxiety is related to the nursing care of patients who are experiencing anxiety.

LEARNING OBJECTIVES

After studying this chapter, the reader will be able to

1. Select the appropriate definitions for anxiety, fear, stress, and crisis.

2. Recognize the causes of and precipitating events associated with anxiety.

3. Recognize the different levels of anxiety.

4. Specify the physiologic responses to anxiety.

5. Recognize the nursing diagnoses pertinent to anxiety.

6. Suggest nursing interventions that may be effective with an anxious patient.

Most patients experience some anxiety about their health. Certainly, hospitalization is a stressor for anyone. Each patient experiences anxiety uniquely and behaves accordingly. If patients cannot cope successfully with their current level of anxiety, helping them regain their coping abilities or use other methods for coping strategically become part of nursing care.

Anxiety is an unpleasant feeling of dread and apprehension. It may be caused by an unconscious conflict between an underlying drive and the reality of the environment, or it may be precipitated by a physical illness or a stressful situation. Anxious persons are often unaware of the specific cause of their feelings.

Fear is an unpleasant feeling caused by the realization and recognition that some event, occurrence, or other detectable source in the environment may bring harm.

Stress, classically described by Hans Selye (1976), is the natural occurrence of wear and tear on the body as the body responds and adapts to life's events. Stress is generally recognized as a highly complex phenomenon. Accordingly, the definition of stress must emphasize the relationship between the person and environment, the situation and the person's physiologic state, the current event and the person's history of stress and coping, and so forth.

Both psychological and physical stress can precipitate feelings of anxiety. These feelings may be successfully coped with in a variety of ways, or they may be overwhelming. When they are overwhelming, the person's coping mechanisms may be insufficient to manage the anxiety.

Crisis is defined as a situation in which a person faces a problem that he or she cannot readily solve by using the coping mechanisms that have worked before (Aguilera, 1990). A crisis is both a danger and an opportunity. It is a danger because of its potential to overwhelm a patient or the patient's family. It is an opportunity because during times of crisis a person is more receptive to therapeutic influence (Aguilera, 1990) and often learns new coping mechanisms. Fortunately, a crisis is a time-limited event.

CAUSES AND PRECIPITATING EVENTS

Some of the causes of anxiety and the precipitating events that lead to it may be unclear or unknown. Almost everyone experiences dread and fear of the unknown. When a person's biological self or self-esteem and self-concept are threatened, feelings of anxiety may arise. Having an illness diagnosed as a dreaded disease or being injured can provoke an identity crisis. In addition to coping with the fear of the disease or injury itself, persons who are ill or injured may have to change their view of themselves.

Everyone goes through maturational stages as part of normal growth and development, and some of these stages can be stressful. Adolescence and old age are typically considered stressful times and may lead to crises. Situational crises also may occur, as people experience various stressful events. Marriage, divorce, having a baby, and losing a loved one are all life events that arouse strong emotions and may precipitate a crisis.

Changes in a person's status are generally stressful. The event can be negative (e.g., an illness) or positive (e.g., the first day on a new job). The precipitating stressors are different for each person.

The culmination of these events and feelings may become a crisis when a person no longer can cope effectively with day-to-day tasks, and normal coping mechanisms fail.

LEVELS OF ANXIETY

Four levels of anxiety are generally recognized:

1. **Mild:** With a mild level of anxiety, a person's ability to cope actually increases. Alertness is increased, and sensory input seems heightened, enabling the person to achieve and succeed in specific tasks.

2. **Moderate:** With a moderate level of anxiety, a person's ability to perceive and communicate is reduced, and a sensation of increased nervousness and tension occurs. Some coping skills are still functional, and the person can follow directions. Therefore, with some help, the anxiety can be dealt with successfully.

3. **Severe:** At the severe level of anxiety, a person's perceptual field becomes quite narrow and focused on the short term. The person's attention span is shortened, and the ability to attend to other things is impaired. An accompanying physical discomfort may add to a sense of emotional discomfort.

4. **Panic:** When anxiety is at the panic level, a person's ability to cope is severely impaired. Perception is distorted. The person has a feeling of terror, and thoughts may be unfocused, random, fleeting, and irrational. A person cannot function at this level for long.

PHYSIOLOGIC RESPONSES

In addition to the many emotional changes that happen when a person is feeling anxious, several physical signs and symptoms may occur. These signs and symptoms are generally experienced negatively.

- Chest pain
- Palpitations
- Dizziness
- Faintness
- Restlessness

- Diaphoresis
- Cold, icy hands
- Trembling
- Dyspnea
- Tachypnea
- Choking or smothering sensations
- Queasiness
- Nausea
- Abdominal distress
- Headaches
- Insomnia
- Fear of dying
- Fear of impending doom

DSM-IV DIAGNOSES

The disorders generally associated with anxiety are as follows:

- Panic disorder with or without agoraphobia
- Obsessive-compulsive disorder
- Posttraumatic stress disorder
- Generalized anxiety disorder

NURSING DIAGNOSES

The nursing diagnoses for anxiety may include one or more of the following:

- Anxiety
- Fear
- Individual coping, ineffective
- Self-care deficit

NURSING INTERVENTIONS

Patients can be helped to cope effectively during times of mild or moderate anxiety by having them use strategies that have been helpful in the past and other problem-solving methods of coping as needed. Patients who are experiencing severe anxiety or panic need help in coping and in reducing the level of anxiety to one at which their problem-solving abilities can be called into play.

The following nursing interventions may be appropriate for patients who are experiencing anxiety:

- **Intervention:** Establish trust, maintain a calm demeanor, and be nonthreatening.

  Rationale: It is well known that anxiety is contagious. A patient's anxiety can affect nurses and staff members and vice versa. The anxious patient needs to rely on someone, and the nurse is an excellent choice.

- **Intervention:** Reassure patients of their safety and security. Staying with the patient, just being there, can be of great value.

  Rationale: Patients may be experiencing a threat to their physical well-being or self-concept.

- **Intervention:** Explore the patient's perception of harm and reality test the potential danger.

  Rationale: Providing reality and assisting with coping mechanisms can reduce anxiety levels.

- **Intervention:** Assess the patient's mood, and observe for signs of depression and any possible suicidal ideation.

  Rationale: Severe anxiety can be a dual diagnosis with depression.

- **Intervention:** Communicate in a calm and clear manner with a succinct message and simple language.

  Rationale: When anxiety levels are high, patients may be unable to comprehend at their usual level of awareness.

- **Intervention:** Assist patients with skills

they currently cannot master because of their anxiety.

Rationale: When anxiety is especially high, usual tasks are more difficult, and learning new tasks is harder.

- **Intervention:** Decrease external stimuli by dimming lights, lowering background noise, and limiting the number and frequency of visitors.

Rationale: External stimuli increase anxiety levels.

- **Intervention:** Administer anxiolytic medications as prescribed, assess the need for medications to be given as needed (prn), assess the effectiveness of the drug, and monitor the patient for potential adverse side effects.

Rationale: Antianxiety medications can be beneficial for short-term use.

- **Intervention:** Teach the patient about the self-administration of anxiolytic medications.

Rationale: The patient may benefit from anxiolytic medications and then continue taking them as an outpatient.

- **Intervention:** When the anxiety level has been reduced, explore the precipitating events.

Rationale: A recurrence of anxiety may be aborted or reduced in severity when the patient can recognize the early signs and can begin using strategies to reduce anxiety.

- **Intervention:** Encourage verbalization.

Rationale: By talking through some events and precipitating factors, patients can gain insight into either the precipitating factor or their manner of coping with the anxiety itself and enact new strategies for coping. Verbalizing one's problems is often helpful in itself.

- **Intervention:** Teach patients the signs and symptoms of anxiety.

Rationale: When patients understand their experience of anxiety, they can recognize the early signs and symptoms and perhaps reduce the level or thwart the episode.

- **Intervention:** Demonstrate and review available anxiety-reducing techniques, and help patients choose techniques and strategies to reduce their anxiety level. These include the following:

  - Relaxation techniques (e.g., breathing techniques, visualization, muscle tension reduction)

  - Physical exercise

  - Meditation and yoga

  - Occupational activity

  - Diversional activity

Rationale: By reducing the level of anxiety, restoration of homeostasis is more obtainable.

- **Intervention:** Include the patient in setting goals and planning care.

Rationale: Allowing patients a choice increases their chances of success and increases their independence and therefore their self-esteem.

CASE STUDY

Robert Bradshaw is a 22-year-old man who was admitted to an orthopedic unit of a general hospital with a fractured femur.

Robert attends a local college. He gets good grades, and he hopes to graduate next June. He is cocaptain of the football team and is considered a star player. He plans to play football professionally after graduation and is considering some offers. His current injury occurred when he was playing football. This is the first time he has had a serious injury.

Robert recently had surgery to treat his injury,

and his left leg is in a cast. He has an intravenous (IV) line and a urinary catheter in place. He is a big man and seems uncomfortable confined to the hospital bed. He has an order for Demerol (meperidine), 75 mg every 4–6 hr prn.

Twenty-four hours after surgery, Robert's nurse notices that he is restless. He calls for the nurse often because of minor complaints and seems to want a nurse in constant contact with him. His requests for pain medications exceed the order, and the night nurse reported that he slept poorly and complained often.

Nurse Boone answers Robert's call-bell light and finds him crying and difficult to console. She approaches him, and he startles her by jumping upright in the bed, pulling at his IV line, and shouting some obscenities. Then he yells, "You just don't get it! This is driving me crazy!" Ms. Boone knows that he is having difficulty adjusting to both his injury and being in the hospital.

She now approaches Robert more quietly. With a soft voice and with a calm demeanor, she asks him to describe what is bothering him. He begins to sob and tells her he is so upset that his ball-playing career has been suspended at this time and that he is worried sick over it.

Ms. Boone correctly recognizes his psychosocial nursing diagnosis and adds problem 5 to his care plan (*Table 3-1*).

Table 3-1
Part of a Care Plan for a Patient with Anxiety

Problem No.   5

Date_____

Problem/Nursing Diagnoses
Anxiety related to change in body image, as evidenced by tension, verbalized and demonstrated helplessness, verbalized fear, uncertainty, expressed concerns, grimacing, perspiration, sobbing, irrational behavior (i.e., pulling at IV, shouting).

Treatment Plan/Approaches
1. Assess level of anxiety.
2. Establish therapeutic relationship.

3. Offer appropriate interventions on the basis of level of anxiety.
- **Mild:** Listen to patient, and redirect activities.
- **Moderate:**
  Consider prn medications if ordered.
  Offer choice between two things.
  Try to decrease stimuli.
  Offer physical activity.
  Use matter-of-fact approach.
- **Severe:** Stay with patient or check him often.
4. Help the patient recognize his feelings and describe what preceded them. If possible, connect the feeling to the unmet need; describe the patient's behavior, and connect it to the anxiety.

EXAM QUESTIONS

CHAPTER 3
Questions 16–23

16–19. Match the levels of anxiety with the following definitions.

   a. Inability to cope

   b. Increased ability to cope

   c. Shortened attention span

   d. Nervousness

16. Mild anxiety — B

17. Moderate anxiety A

18. Severe anxiety C

19. Panic D

20. A threat to a person's self-esteem can do which of the following?

   a. Make the person sick.

   b. Be an event.

   c. Precipitate a major nervous breakdown.

   d. Cause anxiety.

21. Which of the following are physiologic responses to anxiety?

   a. Memory impairment, queasiness

   b. Choking, fatigue

   c. Restlessness, palpitations

   d. Chest pain, decreased pulse rate

22. Establishing trust, maintaining a calm demeanor, and acting in a nonthreatening manner are appropriate nursing interventions for a patient who is which of the following?

   a. Critically ill

   b. Anorectic

   c. Hard of hearing

   d. Anxious

23. Fear, ineffective coping, and self-care deficit are all nursing diagnoses for patients who have which of the following?

   a. Depression

   b. Psychosis

   c. Personality disorder

   d. Anxiety

CHAPTER 4

NURSING MANAGEMENT OF THE PATIENT WITH DEPRESSION OR RELATED MOOD DISORDER

CHAPTER OBJECTIVE

After completing this chapter, the reader will be able to recognize affective illness and how the principles of psychiatric nursing affect the care of a patient with depression or a mood disorder.

LEARNING OBJECTIVES

After studying this chapter, the reader will be able to

1. Correctly define affective illness.

2. Specify the prevalence of depression and the high-risk factors associated with this disorder.

3. Select at least three signs and symptoms of depression.

4. Recognize at least three different theories of causation for depression.

5. Specify disorders associated with depression.

6. Recognize the treatments currently available for depression.

7. Select the correct definition of bipolar affective illness.

8. Recognize the nursing diagnoses related to affective disorders.

9. Indicate which nursing interventions commonly are used with patients with depression.

10. Specify two signs and symptoms of postpartum depression.

DEFINING CHARACTERISTICS

Affective disorder is the name given to a disorder of the internal emotional state of a person that is characterized by (a) extreme sadness, social withdrawal, guilt, and the expression of self-deprecating thoughts or (b) an elevated expansive mood with hyperactivity, pressured speech, decreased need for sleep, and impaired impulse control with poor judgment. The former is usually called a *major affective disorder*; the latter, *bipolar affective disorder*. When a patient's history indicates that both forms occur, the term used is bipolar affective disorder.

DSM-IV DIAGNOSES

The DSM-IV diagnostic categories for depression are listed under the umbrella category of major affective illness. The nurse should find one of the following psychiatric diagnoses among the patient's medical diagnoses in the patient's record:

- **Bipolar affective illness**

  Hypomanic

Manic

Depressed

Mixed

Cyclothymic

- **Major depressive disorder**

Single episode

Recurrent

Dysthymic

PREVALENCE

Sadness...hopelessness...nothing to live for...despair. These sad words describe the feelings of depression. Depression is a disturbance in a person's feelings marked chiefly by sadness, apathy, and loss of energy. An affective illness is a mood disorder. As a disorder, depression is composed of a group of clinical syndromes, the signs and symptoms of which vary somewhat from person to person. Depression can be a common reaction to illness and if prolonged can become maladaptive. Each person's experience of depression is unique; the signs and symptoms are different, and the intensity of the feelings differs. Thus, each person requires individualized interventions.

Depression is the disorder treated most often in psychiatric hospitals today. According to estimates, 25% of people in the United States will become seriously depressed at sometime in their lifetime, and 8 million to 20 million persons currently have depression.

RISK FACTORS

The most serious sequela of depression is suicide. In the United States, suicide rates are 400/100,000 for people with mood disorders and 12.8/100,000 for the general population (Kaplan & Sadock, 1991). According to estimates, approximately 15% of all depressed persons even-

tually succeed with a suicide attempt. The percentage of successful attempts probably is higher, because suicide still carries a stigma, and the reporting of suicides is not always accurate.

An increase in depression is noted in persons more than 60 years old, and the prevalence of depression is generally two times higher in women than in men.

Some of the other high-risk factors for depression include the following:

- Physical illness

- A recent loss of significance (e.g., the death of a family member or friend)

- An event such as a job loss

- Unhappiness with one's life occupation or having no job at all

- Low economic status

- Lack of social networks

- Social isolation

It is important for nonpsychiatric nurses to be aware of the significance of depression among general hospital patients. As many as 24% of all medical patients (i.e., approximately one in four patients) may have a serious depression.

SIGNS AND SYMPTOMS

The signs and symptoms of depression may include the following:

- Depressed mood; feeling sad, empty, or irritable

- Loss of interest or ability to experience pleasure in usual activities

- Low self-esteem, feeling worthless, exaggerated or inappropriate feelings of guilt

- Difficulty thinking or disturbed thought content, ranging from difficulty concentrating and making decisions to the extreme of delusions and hallucinations

- Recurrent thoughts of death or suicidal

ideations, plans, or attempts

- Sleep disturbance: either insomnia, an inability to fall asleep or stay asleep, or hypersomnia, an excessive amount of sleeping

- Psychomotor retardation, feelings of fatigue, withdrawal, and low energy

- Psychomotor agitation with an inability to sit still; continuous pacing and perhaps hand wringing as well

- Appetite disturbance: either a decrease in appetite or overeating and perhaps even binging

- Diminished or no sexual desire

THEORIES OF CAUSATION

Different investigators have different opinions about the causative factors of depression. Some of the more widely known and accepted are the psychosocial and biological theories.

Psychosocial Theories

The psychodynamic or psychoanalytic view is that a loss or lack of love occurred when the person was a young child, and this experience has caused unresolved conflicting feelings and grieving. When these feelings go unresolved, the result may be feelings of rage, hostility, and anger turned inward. Thus, the person becomes depressed.

The cognitive theory, based on the work of Aaron Beck, author of *Cognitive Therapy and the Emotional Disorders* (1976), claims that depressive feelings result from faulty thinking, ideas, and beliefs; a distorted view of others; and a low self-esteem. When the person's thinking or cognition is corrected through cognitive therapy, the depression will be alleviated.

Interpersonal and environmental theories view depression as the result of a breakdown in communication with family, friends, work, school, general activities, and so forth. Individual, group, and family therapies are used in this context.

Biological Theories

Research indicates that depression (as well as other psychiatric disorders) may be due to variations in levels of the biogenic amines. This theory relates to the catecholamines dopamine, norepinephrine, and serotonin and their functioning at their receptor sites on brain cells and nerves.

Genetic factors also play a role in affective disorders. The prevalence of depression and bipolar affective disorders is higher among blood relatives than among the general population: "Approximately 50 percent of all bipolar patients have at least one parent with a mood disorder" (Kaplan & Sadock, 1991).

Of particular note within the context of this book, approximately 10–15% of major depressive episodes are caused by medical illnesses (U.S. Department of Health and Human Services, 1993). Thus, nurses on a general medical-surgical unit must be alert for signs and symptoms of depression in their patients.

Much scientific research is being done in the field of mental illness. Although no definitive cause has been found, more is known about the biological markers of depression now, and treatments are being used successfully.

ASSOCIATED DISORDERS

Some physical and mental illnesses and disorders have a cause-and-effect relationship with depression. The prevalence of depression is generally higher in persons who have concomitant medical problems such as the following:

- **Neurologic disorders**

  Neoplasms

  Stroke

  Multiple sclerosis

  Infections

Trauma

Migraines

- **Endocrine disorders**

  Adrenal disorders

  Thyroid disorders

  Menses-related disorders

  Postpartum disorders

- **Infectious and inflammatory disorders**

  Chronic fatigue syndrome

  Pneumonia

  Acquired immune deficiency syndrome (AIDS)

  Tuberculosis

- **Other medical disorders**

  Vitamin deficiencies

  Anemia

  Cancer

  Cardiopulmonary disease

- **Nonmood psychiatric disorders that often coincide with a diagnosis of depression**

  Obsessive-compulsive disorder

  Panic disorders

  Substance-related disorders

  Personality disorders

  Eating disorders

Depression or mania is an idiosyncratic side effect of many medications, including the following:

- Hypertensive medication (e.g., reserpine)

- Sedatives, tranquilizers, barbiturates, and central nervous system (CNS) depressants

- Steroids (e.g., glucocorticoids, anabolic steroids)

- Cardiac medications

- Hormones (e.g., oral contraceptives)

- Amphetamines, including cocaine and crack, after the effects of these medications wear off

REACTIVE DEPRESSIONS

Some episodes of depression have a clearly detectable precipitating event. Some stressors are difficult for some persons but may not pose problems for others. When assessing patients, the nurse should be aware of the patients' perceptions of their problems as a means of observing for signs and symptoms of depression.

Grief Reaction

Depression can be associated with loss and grief over a loss (i.e., anything a person valued, once had or wanted and now cannot have). This includes losing a spouse, parent, child, other family member, or friend to death or relocation. Situational grieving associated with events such as losing a job, divorce, and financial losses commonly are associated with a short-term depression.

Trauma

Some form of disaster or physical trauma, such as an accidental injury or a major illness, can precipitate an episode of depression.

Postpartum Blues

Postpartum depressions and postpartum psychosis are two of the psychiatric disorders that may affect a woman shortly after she gives birth. Studies have shown that 20–40% of new mothers experience some emotional disturbance during the postpartum period (Kaplan & Sadock, 1991). In addition to hormonal shifts, inner psychological conflicts can occur over becoming a mother for the first time, or once again.

The severity of signs and symptoms varies. Some new mothers may experience sleep disturbances, increased anxiety, fatigue, irritability, or negative or ambivalent emotions toward and about the baby. Less often, the new mother has a full-blown psychosis. She may be profoundly depressed and suicidal, hallucinating or delusional, having homicidal thoughts or unreal feelings about the child (e.g., that the child is sick or dead). The psychotic episodes seem to occur in 1–2 births per 1,000 (Kaplan & Sadock, 1991).

Symptoms generally occur 3 days after the birth and usually within the first week. Some of the more minor symptoms may be present in various degrees from 1 month to 1 year. Because of the short times new mothers stay in most maternity units and birthing centers, nurses working on those units may not see the full extent of these disorders. Extreme or dangerous situations may result in the patient being readmitted, but usually to a psychiatric service. In the absence of life-threatening crises, attempts generally are made to care for patients at home. The patient can have continuity in bonding and mothering the newborn, the comfort of a familiar environment, and, it is hoped, family support.

Baby blues are a minor form of postpartum depression that occurs in up to 50% of all new mothers (Kaplan & Sadock, 1991). New mothers may be irritable, anorectic, easily fatigued yet unable to sleep, and crying a lot. Fortunately, these episodes are usually self-limiting, lasting only a few days. However, the frequency of these signs and symptoms is high enough to warrant giving the new mother bedside education about them while she is in the maternity unit. Nurses working in the community who may see new mothers in the mothers' homes a week or more after the birth should be alert to the signs and symptoms of baby blues and its equivalent psychiatric disorder.

TREATMENT OPTIONS

Different types of treatments are used for patients with depression, and consideration is given to the patient's history and severity of signs and symptoms. In general, a combination of some form of psychotherapy and an antidepressant medication is the preferred treatment.

Psychotherapies

Psychotherapy is used in both inpatient and outpatient settings, on short- and long-term bases. Patients may be treated individually, within groups, or with family members. Scientific evidence indicates that several forms of short-term psychotherapy (cognitive, interpersonal, and behavioral) are effective in treating most cases of mild or moderate depression (U.S. Dept. of Health and Human Services, 1993). Treatments are based on a variety of theories, such as systems theory, communications theory, and interpersonal theory.

Somatic Treatments

Psychopharmacologic therapy. Since the 1960s, the use of tricyclic antidepressants and monoamine oxidase inhibitors in combination with psychotherapy has constituted the principal mode of treatment. In the past several years, selective serotonin reuptake inhibitors have become available.

With estimated efficacy rates of 70–80%, psychopharmacologic therapy is a popular form of treatment of depression. Newer drugs, such as the selective serotonin reuptake inhibitors, work faster and produce fewer side effects and thus are becoming the first-line drugs of choice. Generally, tricyclic antidepressants take 2–3 weeks to produce therapeutic results.

Electroconvulsive therapy. Electroconvulsive therapy (ECT) is an effective treatment for depression. The patient is anesthetized, and a seizure is induced. Treatments are given in a series of 6–10 over 2–3 weeks. ECT is primarily indicated for severe depressions and bipolar affective disorder. Although the short-term memory loss associated with this type of therapy is well-known, more profound and longer lasting adverse effects are rare. When appropriately administered, ECT is an effective choice in the treatment and alleviation of depression.

BIPOLAR AFFECTIVE ILLNESS

Bipolar affective illness (formerly called manic-depressive illness) is an affective illness in which the person experiences episodes of mania or hypomania (less intense form of mania) that alternate with bouts of depression. The severity of signs and symptoms in each episode varies from person to person.

Evidence is strong that some heredity factors are involved. Persons with bipolar affective illness usually can trace a family pattern of this disturbance. Approximately 50% of all patients with bipolar affective illness have at least one parent with a mood disorder (Kaplan & Sadock, 1991).

Signs and Symptoms of Mania or Hypomania

The signs and symptoms of mania or hypomania include the following:

- Euphoria, grandiosity
- Feeling irritable, easily disturbed, destractible
- Increased talkativeness; rapid, pressured speech; flight of ideas with racing thoughts
- Decreased need for sleep, physical restlessness
- Hypersexuality, perhaps promiscuousness
- Poor judgment, often with impulsive behavior
- Delusional thoughts and possibly hallucinations
- Psychomotor agitation

For many persons who have bipolar affective illness, lithium carbonate is effective in the management and stabilization of the illness. Patients who are taking lithium carbonate must have their serum levels of the drug monitored closely. The medication must be taken continuously; its effectiveness is contingent on maintaining a certain level in the blood.

Nursing Diagnoses for Depression and Bipolar Affective Illness

Nursing diagnoses for depression and bipolar affective illness may include one or more of the following:

- Dysfunctional grieving
- Social isolation
- Individual coping, ineffective
- Powerlessness
- Altered nutrition
- Sleep pattern disturbance
- Thought processes, altered
- Sensory or perceptual alterations: auditory
- Risk for injury
- Risk for violence, self-directed or directed at others
- Anxiety
- Hopelessness

NURSING INTERVENTIONS

Patient in a general hospital may experience a primary or secondary mood disorder. Patients with depression or mania may be receiving treatment for the disorder before or during their hospital stay. Nurses who administer care at the bedside can provide valuable assistance to these patients by using some of the following nursing interventions. Because they spend so much time with patients, nurses are in a strategically important place for assessing a patient's mood and making an appropriate referral for treatment.

- **Intervention:** Be accepting. The patient may have a negative outlook and low self-esteem.

  Rationale: An attitude of acceptance enhances feelings of self-worth.

- **Intervention:** Be nonjudgmental, develop a trusting relationship, and be open with the patient.

Rationale: Trust is basic to a therapeutic relationship.

- **Intervention:** Encourage verbalization of problems, as seen by the patient (e.g., grieving a loss, internal mood, isolation, dysfunctional thinking).

Rationale: If patients recognize possible precipitating events, they can take steps to reduce occurrence of the events or to devise strategies that may reduce or eliminate the stressors.

- **Intervention:** Encourage patients to make their own choices when they experience feelings of powerlessness.

Rationale: Patients gain a sense of control and mastery when they make choices.

- **Intervention:** Check the patient often.

Rationale: Depressed patients need short frequent contacts to assure them that they are supported, safe, and attended to, even when they may feel that they are not worth your attention.

- **Intervention:** If the patient has experienced a loss, describe the stages of grieving and teach the patient about them.

Rationale: Knowledge of the process of normal grieving helps patients accept their own feelings.

- **Intervention:** Allow the patient to cry in a supportive environment.

Rationale: Crying helps the patient relieve pent-up feelings.

- **Intervention:** Help the patient determine appropriate ways of expressing anger.

Rationale: Patients with a moderate amount of depression are often angry. Patients who are have bipolar affective illness are often unstable and angry.

- **Intervention:** Assess the patient for suicidal ideation, and initiate safety checks and procedures as indicated.

Rationale: Patients with depression may have suicidal feelings and thoughts.

- **Intervention:** Assess the patient for any indications of a thought disorder.

Rationale: Some patients with depression have an accompanying thought disorder, and there can be a cause-and-effect relationship between the two. Patients who have depression or bipolar affective disorder may have psychotic thoughts.

- **Intervention:** Assist the patient in problem solving.

Rationale: Problem solving reduces stresses and increases the patient's self-esteem.

- **Intervention:** Encourage the patient to participate in an available or appropriate group.

Rationale: The patient may receive positive feedback as well as feel supported. Patients are often more open to what other patients suggest.

- **Intervention:** Encourage patients to increase their interpersonal contacts.

Rationale: Interpersonal relationships can reduce feelings of social isolation.

- **Intervention:** Assess the patient's ability to perform self-care tasks.

Rationale: Depression may decrease a person's ability to continue usual activities of daily living.

- **Intervention:** Assess the patient's sleep patterns and determine methods to either reduce or increase sleep. Methods to reduce hypersomnia include increasing stimulation, keeping well occupied, and socializing. Methods to promote sleep include using relaxation techniques, exercising earlier in the day, decreasing stimulation at rest time, and drinking warm milk.

Rationale: Disturbances in sleep patterns are common in patients with depression or bipolar affective disorder. Avoiding hypersomnia and successfully alleviating insomnia help patients recover from their affective illness.

- **Intervention:** Administer antidepressant medications as prescribed. Assess the effectiveness of the medication, and monitor the patient for potential side effects.

  Rationale: Antidepressant medications are an effective treatment for depression.

- **Intervention:** Teach the patient about the self-administration of antidepressant medications.

  Rationale: Although quite beneficial for many patients, antidepressant medications are quite potent and must be monitored carefully.

- **Intervention:** Assist with the administration of ECT on an inpatient or outpatient basis. Provide nursing care to the patient who has received ECT.

  Rationale: ECT is safe and effective in the treatment of depression.

- **Intervention:** On a home visit or outpatient clinic or office visit, monitor the effects and side effects of treatment for patients who have had ECT.

  Rationale: If unsupervised, patients treated with ECT may be unsafe because of pronounced confusion. The continued need for treatments is based on the patient's response.

- **Intervention:** Reduce the environmental stimuli for patients experiencing a hypomanic or manic episode.

  Rationale: Patients are generally quite easily distracted when they are manic.

- **Intervention:** Provide structure and set limits as guides for a manic patient.

  Rationale: Generally, manic patients show poor judgment and impulsivity; they may need guidance.

- **Intervention:** Assess the patient for possible injury; ensure the patient's safety.

  Rationale: Patients may need protection from harm.

- **Intervention:** Provide the patient an opportunity to express pent-up emotions; use appropriate physical activities if the patient can be mobile.

  Rationale: Physical activity can reduce tension.

- **Intervention:** Administer lithium carbonate if indicated, and teach patients about the medication and the need for monitoring lithium levels.

  Rationale: Lithium carbonate is effective and potent. Patients generally require this medication long term and will need to have levels monitored regularly.

- **Intervention:** Administer tranquilizers if indicated.

  Rationale: Some manic episodes that are extreme and that may cause a patient harm may be reduced by the short-term use of a tranquilizer to help the patient maintain a sense of equilibrium and homeostasis.

CASE STUDY

Mrs. Lenox is a 47-year-old woman who was admitted to a surgical unit of a general hospital and had an ovarian cyst removed. The procedure went well, and medically Mrs. Lenox is doing fine.

Ms. Hill, the evening nurse, was with the patient and noted that Mrs. Lenox seemed depressed. The patient and her husband divorced last year. Her second child, a daughter, left for college in the past 2 months, and her oldest child, a son, is married and living 500 miles away. Mrs. Lenox admitted that she has been feeling sad, having frequent crying spells, having a poor appetite, and being more tired than usual. She claims that she falls asleep easily at about 11 p.m. each night but finds herself wide awake at 2 a.m., unable to return to sleep and feeling quite dreadful.

Ms. Hill accurately diagnoses the problem as depression and over the course of the next few days does the following:

- Discusses what she thinks with Mrs. Lenox.

- Teaches Mrs. Lenox the signs and symptoms of depression.

- Discusses her findings with Mrs, Lenox's physician, who agrees.

- Sends a referral for professional psychiatric assessment.

- Makes additional time to spend with Mrs. Lenox, encouraging verbalization.

- Observes for changes in behaviors that had been indications of the patient's depression: saddened face, crying spells, feelings of dread, poor appetite, and early morning awakening.

SUMMARY

Depression is an affective illness seen regularly in the general hospital. When nurses accurately assess this problem, steps can be taken to ensure that the patient receives appropriate treatment while in the hospital and after discharge.

Patients in the general hospital who have bipolar affective illness may be taking medication to control the disorder. Such patients must be monitored during their stay and observed for any changes in behavior.

Nursing interventions for patients who have an affective illness are quite effective in helping the patients maintain a psychosocial balance while in the hospital and perhaps in helping them take steps for ongoing care.

EXAM QUESTIONS

CHAPTER 4
Questions 24–33

24. For a patient who has experienced a loss, describing the stages of grieving and teaching the patient about them are nursing interventions for which of the following problems?

    a. Psychosis

    b. Confusion and organicity

    c. Depression

    d. Loss of control

25–29. True or false, the following are signs or symptoms of depression.

    a. True

    b. False

25. Inability to experience pleasure in usual activities T

26. Anorexia T

27. Agranulocytosis F

28. Low self-esteem T

29. Uncontrollable laughter F

30. Bipolar affective illness is which of the following?

    a. A life-threatening illness

    b. Baby blues

    c. An affective illness with bouts of highs and lows

    d. A reactive depression

31. Interpersonal theorists view depression as which of the following?

    a. An incomplete cognition

    b. A biochemical imbalance

    c. A breakdown in communication with family and friends

    d. The result of an event in childhood

32. Which of the following is the treatment of choice for a patient with severe persistent depression who is dangerously suicidal?

    a. Long-term analytic treatment

    b. Electroconvulsive therapy

    c. Crisis intervention

    d. Antipsychotic medications

33. Which of the following is included in the nursing diagnoses for a patient with depression?

    a. Alteration in mood

    b. Affective illness

    c. Risk for self-directed violence

    d. Alteration in affect

CHAPTER 5

NURSING MANAGEMENT OF THE SUICIDAL PATIENT

CHAPTER OBJECTIVE

After completing this chapter, the reader will be able to assess suicidal ideation in a patient and specify which nursing interventions may be useful in caring for such a patient.

LEARNING OBJECTIVES

After studying this chapter, the reader will be able to

1. Recognize some facts about the prevalence of suicide in the United States.

2. Specify two of the theories of causation for suicide attempts.

3. Select two high-risk factors for predicting suicidal ideation.

4. Indicate two false beliefs nurses may have about persons who attempt suicide.

5. Specify three variables of a lethality assessment.

6. Recognize the nursing diagnoses related to the suicidal patient.

7. Indicate which nursing interventions commonly are used with patients who have suicidal ideation.

OVERVIEW OF THE PROBLEM

Suicide is the most common serious sequela of the mental and emotional disorders. It is the consequence of a successfully executed, self-directed violent act. The suicidal person may be any age, male or female, rich or poor. No culture is immune, and no race or religion is protected. Suicide is the final and most drastic step toward attempting to cope, manage, or deal with one or more perceived threats to the self, whether they be biological, psychological, or emotional.

Accurate data and statistics on the rate of suicide are difficult to gather because suicide continues to be veiled by stigma. Some suicides are not reported, and some causes of death are recorded inaccurately. People who commit suicide finally succumb to their illness, but there is no finality for the survivors, that is, friends, relatives, and acquaintances.

According to estimates, each year 30,000–40,000 persons in the United States make a successful suicide attempt. Although more women than men attempt suicide, men are more often successful, probably because men use more lethal means (McFarland & Thomas, 1991). Since 1985, the number of suicides among adolescents and young adults 15–24 years old has increased, but consistently the number is highest for the elderly. As many as 25% of suicides, or one in four, is a person more than 65 years old.

Staff nurses in the general hospital may come into contact with a suicidal person in a variety of ways. Some patients who are unsuccessful in their suicide attempt may be hospitalized as a consequence of a shooting, cutting, carbon monoxide poisoning, or overdose. The patients who survive a suicide attempt often are brought to a general hospital emergency department, where they receive medical treatment before or at the same time as their psychiatric treatment. Patients in the general hospital often are depressed, and they may attempt suicide even while in the hospital.

Nurses who work in outpatient settings, clinics, offices, or home care may discover a patient's suicidal wishes or face the outcome of a failed attempt. A general hospital nurse may initially assess and triage these patients.

Persons with thoughts of harming themselves may be overwhelmed by unbearable emotions. Persons who are suicidal may have distorted thinking. They may be psychotic or confused or under the influence of drugs or alcohol. Persons who have serious medical problems with severe pain or a terminal illness may see no other way out for themselves and may think of suicide as a release.

Depressed persons experience emotions such as the following:

- Despair
- Guilt
- Shame
- Hopelessness
- Helplessness
- Extreme weariness

Sometimes they feel as though life is no longer worth living because they find no meaning in their own existence. Some people with multiple problems have few or no coping skills and cannot see any solutions to the problems. Other suicidal persons feel an overwhelming sense of responsibility for someone else's unhappiness (e.g., a spouse, parent, or child) and think this other person would be better off without them. Whatever the person's situation, the emotions are generally deep and overwhelming.

THEORIES OF CAUSATION

Suicide is not a new phenomenon. Although each person's situation is unique, several theories of causation have been formulated. A review of the situations of those who have attempted suicide gives an understanding of the depth of the problem. Suicide attempts and gestures must always be taken seriously and considered a call for help. People who are suicidal may be unable to articulate their feelings, may feel unheard, or may know no other way to call attention to themselves and the situation.

In the rational theory, suicide is considered a result of trying to escape from a painful life situation, perhaps an illness or a major loss. The person may be grief stricken because of the death of a spouse, a life partner, or a child. The men who jumped from high Wall Street windows in New York City in the famous stock market crash of 1929 were experiencing tremendous financial losses and probably felt deep humiliation, defeat, and impending doom.

Some credence is given to the theory that suicide is really murder turned inward. According to this theory, the suicidal person feels deeply aggressive. He or she has murderous thoughts about someone else but is unable to act on this rage toward another. Finding no other solution to these overwhelming feelings, the person commits suicide. A related idea is that the only way suicidal persons can gain some control over themselves or their particular situation is to kill themselves, thereby showing some mastery over their own fate.

RISK FACTORS

Although no definite means are available to predict who may attempt suicide, a number of precipitating factors are associated with many suicides and therefore are considered high-risk factors. These include the following:

- Chemical dependency, alcoholism, and other substance abuse

- Pain in those who are severely medically ill, with chronic or terminal disease

- Recent catastrophic loss

- Major psychiatric illness: depression, schizophrenia, or anxiety disorders

- Cumulative losses

FALSE BELIEFS

Although it is almost impossible to predict who will commit suicide, some widespread myths about suicide exist. A common myth is that people who talk about suicide will never actually kill themselves. This belief is generally the opposite of what really happens. Most people who attempt suicide do talk about their suicidal feelings or give clues about their despondency. According to estimates, this group includes approximately 80% of successful suicides. Most suicidal persons have some ambivalence and feel a need to express feelings of despair and confusion.

Some medical personnel believe that a suicide threat is just a means to get some attention. Although it is true that a suicide attempt is a cry for help, each person's mind is complex, and all suicidal threats should be taken seriously. Some nurses think that they will plant suicidal ideas into the brain of a distraught person by merely mentioning or asking about suicide during an interaction or assessment. This belief is absolutely false. If a nurse thinks a patient may be suicidal, assessment of the patient must include direct questions about suicide.

ASSESSMENT

Patients who are thought to be suicidal need careful monitoring and assessment of their suicidal potential. If a nurse thinks a patient may be suicidal, the nurse should ask. This can be phrased in many ways:

- Are you thinking of killing yourself?

- Have you been considering ways to harm yourself?

- Do you feel like hurting yourself?

- Do you mean you are feeling suicidal?

- Have you been thinking of hurting yourself?

Sometimes patients leave guarded or veiled messages, perhaps a note or a letter. Suicidal patients may suddenly give away valuable property, such as jewelry, inappropriately. Markedly depressed patients who suddenly seem "better" may have made a decision to kill themselves. They feel relieved by deciding to do so and thereby take some action. The nurse may discover that they have telephoned others to say good-bye.

Although no absolute predictive measures are available, a careful assessment can provide enough information so that attempts to protect the patient can be made immediately and long-term assistance can be sought for them. The following variables make up a *lethality assessment* that can help determine which patients are at high risk for suicide.

Risk Factors

Does the patient have some of the high-risk factors mentioned before, such as serious medical or psychiatric illness? Are they chemically dependent? Have they experienced a recent loss?

Demographics

Age, sex, and race should be considered.

Statistics show that elderly people and whites are more likely than younger people or nonwhites to commit suicide, and more men than women succeed at suicide, although more women attempt it. Suicide has a high prevalence among 15- to 24-year-olds and among 20- to 35-year-old black, urban men. These young age groups are less likely than other age groups to be seen in a general hospital. More single people than married people attempt suicide.

Social Factors

The prevalence of suicide is high among persons who are socially isolated, withdrawn, or independent and among persons with little or no religious affiliation. Some religions hold strict beliefs against suicide. They consider suicide a sin, and this belief may make a difference in a pious person. Suicide also occurs more often among the unemployed, those forced to retire, young people from broken homes, and those whose families are in discord.

Resources

Does the patient have any family, friends, community organizations, or groups of any sort that they are attached to or affiliated with? Is the patient in communication with others on a regular basis? These factors may be helpful in discouraging suicidal thoughts.

Personal History

Has the person attempted suicide in the past? If so, how many times, how often, and how lethal the method? People who have attempted suicide before and are again in crisis are more likely to attempt suicide again. Has a family member committed suicide? Having a history of a family member or close friend commit suicide increases a person's risk for self-inflicted death.

Plan

If a patient admits to being suicidal, it is crucial to determine the patient's plan. Does the patient have a plan? If so, what is it? Is the patient imminently at risk in the hospital? Is the patient thinking of jumping from a high hospital window or of using a knife or other sharp instrument? For example, one man who had had open heart surgery cut his neck with a small penknife in the middle of the night while he was on the recovery unit. He had hidden the knife under his pillow and had been despondent over the loss of his wife, who had died 6 months earlier. Other patients may be thinking of shooting themselves, but they do not have a gun. Others may be thinking of taking a lethal overdose of medications and either have the drugs in their possession or are storing up the medication by not swallowing the doses as given.

The nurse needs to assess not only the potential means but also the availability of immediate access to complete the plan. Generally speaking, guns are the most lethal method, and drug overdoses the least. The danger of a patient succeeding is less imminent if the plan is to jump off a bridge or drown in the ocean. Obviously, these methods are not easily accessible to patients in the general hospital (Burgess, 1990).

NURSING DIAGNOSES

Two nursing diagnoses are directly related to the suicidal act:

1. Risk for violence: self-directed
2. Hopelessness

Other nursing diagnoses are relevant to each person's precipitating problems, for example, diagnoses related to the person's inability to cope, grief, or overwhelming feelings of depression.

NURSING INTERVENTIONS

The following nursing interventions can be used with a patient who is actually or potentially suicidal.

- **Intervention:** Assess the patient's suicidal intent. Ask the patient outright about suicide. Always take threats of suicide seriously and assess the imminent lethality potential. Determine how dangerous the patient can be. Continually assess the patient's impulse control.

  Rationale: Once a correct assessment is made of the patient's suicidal ideation, steps can be taken to ensure the patient's safety.

- **Intervention:** Create a safe environment. The patient should be visible, within eyesight of staff members, or checked often or monitored by using some system in which staff members are accountable for the patient's whereabouts. Perhaps the patient needs one-on-one care or monitoring whereby he or she is with a staff member, at arms length and in full view, at all times. Medications should be taken in the presence of a nurse, and the patient should be checked for "cheeking" (not swallowing the pills, holding them in a corner of the mouth). The patient's property should be examined, and any potentially dangerous objects (e.g., glass, razor, scissors, knives, belts) should be removed.

  Rationale: Treatment can be sought or begun while the patient is protected from self-harm.

- **Intervention:** Establish a therapeutic relationship with the patient. Spend time with the patient. Encourage expression of feelings and verbalization of thoughts.

  Rationale: The patient may experience an increase in self-esteem, feel safe, and feel some relief from overwhelming thoughts and feelings.

- **Intervention:** Make a verbal behavioral contract with the patient that includes the expectation that the patient will not harm himself or herself and will seek out staff members to verbalize suicidal feelings.

  Rationale: Most suicidal patients experience ambivalence and can be prompted into remaining safe by have them "give their word" to follow through on the safety contract.

- **Intervention:** Help the patient use effective coping methods. Help the patient use a problem-solving approach, with a focus on short-term resolution of the problem.

  Rationale: Suicidal patients often feel unable to see other ways out and need to build their way into the future.

- **Intervention:** Help the patient assess his or her strengths and weaknesses. Help him or her recognize actual resources, both personal and social, and potential ones not yet considered.

  Rationale: When coping methods are increased, solutions to some of life's problems can be attained.

- **Intervention:** If the patient is cognitively impaired, evaluate the patient's mental status and institute reality testing along with reorientation.

  Rationale: Patients can be protected from inadvertently and unintentionally harming themselves as a result of a thought disorder.

- **Intervention:** Provide nursing management for any possible sequelae from an unsuccessful suicide attempt, (e.g., an aborted shooting, cutting, hanging, overdose, poisoning).

  Rationale: Emergency medical care needs to be instituted for life support.

- **Intervention:** Notify and alert appropriate

caregivers about the risk for suicide and the plan of care.

Rationale: Appropriate communication to other caregivers and consistency in approach will be helpful.

- **Intervention:** Make referrals for immediate and long-term discharge needs.

Rationale: The reason for the patient's suicidal ideation should be diagnosed and treated. The patient should be monitored continually until he or she is no longer suicidal.

EXAM QUESTIONS

CHAPTER 5
Questions 34–38

34. Murder turned inward refers to which of the following?

    a. Rage

    b. A violent assault

    c. A causative theory of suicide

    d. An untoward incident

35. A suicide attempt is often precipitated by which of the following?

    a. A telephone call

    b. Ingestion of a chemical substance

    c. A major loss

    d. A manic episode

36. What percentage of people who commit suicide previously talked about killing themselves or gave clues about their despondency?

    a. 25%

    b. 40%

    c. 55%

    d. 80%

37. Which of the following factors are considered during a lethality assessment?

    a. The patient's education

    b. The patient's coping resources and suicide plan

    c. The patient's marital status and number of children

    d. The patient's physical endurance and future goals

38. What nursing intervention is most important when working with a suicidal patient?

    a. Provide support and reassurance.

    b. Teach stress management.

    c. Change the patient's wound dressing.

    d. Create a safe environment.

CHAPTER 6

NURSING MANAGEMENT OF THE PSYCHOTIC PATIENT

CHAPTER OBJECTIVE

After completing this chapter, the reader will be able to recognize psychosis in a patient and intervene appropriately.

LEARNING OBJECTIVES

After studying this chapter, the reader will be able to

1. Correctly define psychosis.

2. Specify the five types of hallucinations.

3. Recognize three types of delusions.

4. Recognize three signs or symptoms of psychosis.

5. Specify one altered mechanism of speech that a psychotic patient may have.

6. Indicate two possible causes of psychosis.

7. Specify the nursing diagnoses related to psychosis.

8. Select three factors important to consider when making a nursing assessment of a psychotic patient.

9. Recognize the nursing interventions that can be used for a patient who is psychotic.

BACKGROUND AND DEFINITIONS

The most severe signs and symptoms of psychosis are the aberrant behaviors that many people label as "crazy." Persons who are experiencing hallucinations and suffering from delusions constitute a fair percentage of patients on psychiatric wards. Patients who are psychotic often are feared and shunned when they are cared for by personnel who are not knowledgeable mental health professionals. Generally, psychotic persons are not dangerous; however, because their thinking is irrational, their behavior may be irrational also and can therefore be unpredictable.

People may be psychotic for a variety of medical and psychiatric reasons. These include brain disorders, reactions to some medications, and biochemical disturbances. Usually, a general hospital nurse can expect to work with patients who are psychotic acutely and briefly because of some organic cause.

Persons with schizophrenia may be psychotic periodically throughout the duration of their illness. The signs and symptoms and the severity of different episodes of psychosis vary. People who have schizophrenia or other psychiatric illnesses sometimes require treatment in general hospitals and may require specialized and thoughtful nursing care for both their medical and their psychiatric problems.

Psychosis can be defined broadly as a mental state in which a person may exhibit delusions, hallucinations, disorganized speech, grossly disorganized or catatonic behavior, or a gross impairment in reality testing (Kaplan & Sadock, 1991). The two most severe indications of psychosis are hallucinations and delusions.

HALLUCINATIONS

A *hallucination* is false sensory input. Hallucinations may take different forms:

- **Auditory:** Hearing voices or noises that are not truly present, by far the most common form of hallucinations. Examples include hearing a dead family member speak and hearing the voice of God or the devil.

- **Visual:** Seeing things that are not there. Examples are seeing bats flying around the room and seeing bugs crawling on the ground.

- **Olfactory:** Smelling strange, different or unique odors (generally the patient is preoccupied by them). Examples are foul body odors, animal odors, "the smell of disease," and some caustic chemical smell or odor.

- **Gustatory:** Having a bad (i.e., strange, perhaps foul and nauseating) taste in the mouth, sometimes associated with eating or drinking something. An example is drinking something that tastes like "poison or blood."

- **Tactile:** Having things feel strange to the touch or having strange bodily sensations (e.g., bugs crawling on the body); experiencing objects as feeling odd and different.

All forms of hallucinations can vary in their severity; some are mild and some are severe. The amount of cognitive impairment that causes the hallucination or the functioning that results from hallucinations varies from person to person and may even be different in each episode for each person.

DELUSIONS

A *delusion* is a distortion in thinking in which a person has a fixed false belief that usually involves a misperception of reality. Delusions generally follow some theme.

- **Grandeur:** An inflated belief in one's self-importance or believing that one is someone prominent (who may be dead or alive), such as Jesus Christ, God, Napoleon, or Joan of Arc.

- **Persecution:** A dreadful sense of being followed, pursued, or threatened by others in a harmful manner. A person might believe that the Federal Bureau of Investigation, the Central Intelligence Agency, or the Mafia "is out to get me."

- **Reference:** A belief that environmental events and situations or other persons' behavior has a special relationship to the patient, sometimes in a controlling manner. Examples are seeing two people holding hands as a message that the patient will never experience a love relationship and receiving coded messages from the television or radio.

- **Somatic delusion:** A false sense of how one's body is functioning. For example, a perfectly healthy woman "knows" that she is dying from cancer that is rampant in her body.

OTHER SIGNS AND SYMPTOMS

Psychotic persons may exhibit any number of strange and bizarre behaviors. Aside from these, the manner of communication can be indicative of altered thinking. Not only the way persons speak but also the process and content of what they say may show strong evidence of psychosis.

Some of the signs and symptoms of psychosis are as follows:

- **Inappropriate affect:** What is the appearance of the patient's face? Is the patient laughing at some tragic news or crying about something funny? Does the way the patient appear match appropriately the context of the situation and the content of speech?

- **Regression:** Some patients with long psychiatric histories seem quite dependent and needy; they behave in a childlike manner.

- **Hyperreligiosity:** Some patients seem overly religious. They are involved fervently with the church, God, and the Bible, often to the exclusion of all else. Sometimes the religious persuasion is questionable, and the beliefs may seem to be of a delusional proportion to reality.

- **Concrete thinking:** The patient takes things said literally. Persons with schizophrenia or developmental retardation think in this primitive manner.

- **Looseness of associations:** The patient connects random thoughts and experiences in a loose and perhaps strange way and does not make much sense.

- **Strange mechanisms of speech:** Patients who are psychotic, especially those who are schizophrenic, may use odd patterns of speech. These include *echolalia,* repeating what another person says; *neologisms,* making up new words that have hidden meanings and then using the new words in the course of conversation, thinking others understand them; and *word salad,* using a jumble of mixed-up words in a sentence.

CAUSATIVE FACTORS

A psychosis may be acute or chronic, and it may be the sequela of organic or functional disorders. As previously mentioned, in the general hospital, psychoses associated with psychiatric illness are seen less often than those associated with medical or organic illnesses. Psychiatric disorders that may have some psychotic features include the following:

- **Schizophrenia:** Schizophrenia is a disorder with multiple psychological impairments that commonly include psychosis.

- **Affective disorders:** Persons with severe depression and some with bipolar affective illness may experience psychotic thinking.

- **Personality disorders:** Some persons who have a severe disturbance of personality may have episodes of disordered thinking and exhibit psychotic thinking. The personality disorders are included in the DSM-IV *(see the appendix).*

Some persons in the midst of a crisis have disordered thought processes and may become transiently psychotic. A patient in a general care hospital or one who is undergoing some sort of medical crisis, physically and psychologically, may experience a crisis. This detail should not be overlooked when an assessment is done.

As with patients who are in a crisis, patients who are sensory deprived or overstimulated have an increase in stress and thus can become psychotic. Many hospital intensive care units (ICUs) use the terms *ICU psychosis* and *ICU-itis.* This condition is thought to be a result of simply being a patient in an ICU and experiencing an overabundance of noise, odors, and the physical procedures done by so many physicians, nurses, and technicians throughout the day and night.

The organic causes of psychosis are more easily defined. Such psychoses are generally short term, unless they stem specifically from a chronic illness. Organic causes include the following:

- **Brain dysfunction:** Either brain damage from an assault or trauma or a brain disorder associated with some disease or lesion can cause psychosis. Some patients with organic brain disorders, including patients with delirium or dementia, may become psychotic. High fevers, acute infections, and systemic illness can cause psychosis.

- **Toxic substances:** A toxic response to various substances and medications can induce psychosis. Some medications, such as levodopa, can cause psychosis. With others, such as steroids, withdrawal from the medication can cause psychosis. Drug abusers can become psychotic. For some drugs (such as with LSD, PCP, mescaline, and the hallucinogens), the cause of the psychosis is the drug's specific action. High doses of other drugs, such as crystal methamphetamine, other amphetamines, cocaine, and crack, can induce psychoses. Alcoholic delirium or delirium tremens, the severe sign of withdrawal from alcohol, may include psychosis. As with any toxic or foreign substance, any specific drug can have an adverse effect on someone, either during the period of intoxication or in the withdrawal phase.

NURSING DIAGNOSES

The following nursing diagnoses may be relevant to a patient who is psychotic:

- Altered thought processes
- Sensory or perceptual alteration: auditory or visual
- Impaired verbal communication
- Ineffective individual coping
- Risk for violence: self-directed or directed at others

ASSESSMENT

Nursing assessment of the psychotic patient should include a mental status examination. Describe the exact nature of the patient's psychosis. Interview the patient, and document the evidence of psychotic communication and thinking. The interview may elicit bizarre and strange remarks and behaviors. Document these responses by citing direct quotes from the patient and giving specifics of any unusual mannerisms, dress, or behaviors.

Observe the patient closely. Persons who are seeing things or hearing voices may be looking vacant or may be attentive to something that is not obvious to you. Psychotic persons appear watchful and apprehensive. Look for excessive signs of stress, tension, and agitation. Persons who are hallucinating or are delusional may seem quite internally preoccupied or distractible. They may seem to have difficulty understanding you and following your conversation. They may mumble or talk to themselves. They may use socially unacceptable speech, cursing, and erratic tones of voice. Check the patient's history for previous psychiatric disorders, and report the psychosis to the patient's physician and related health care providers.

Once the cause of the patient's psychosis has been determined, treatment can be begun, and planning for long-term care can be considered. Most psychoses seen in the general hospital are associated with some acute medically related event, disorder, or substance. Treatment of these psychoses is generally effective.

NURSING INTERVENTIONS

The following nursing interventions can be used for patients who are psychotic:

- **Intervention:** Provide a safe environment. Check the patient's potential for self-harm or harm to others. Observe the patient often.

  Rationale: Psychotic patients can be distraught enough to attempt suicide. Command hallucinations, voices that tell a person to harm himself or herself, are extremely dangerous to the patient's safety.

Persons who are delusional and feel persecuted may act out violently, irrationally, and impulsively toward others.

- **Intervention:** Decrease stimulation.

  Rationale: If the patient is overly excited or responding to a great deal of anxiety, creating a more relaxing, restful, and calming atmosphere may decrease the entire episode or the intensity of the psychosis.

- **Intervention:** Establish rapport and a trusting relationship. Make brief but frequent contacts with the patient. Approach the patient with acceptance and a nonthreatening manner.

  Rationale: These measures provide support and reassurance.

- **Intervention:** Do not argue with psychotic patients. Let them know you believe them, that they are in fact reporting the truth as they know it. Tell them the reality from your perspective. Remind them of time, place, and person. You may want to say, "I know you are fearful of being harmed by aliens, but there is no evidence of their presence here now," or "I don't see any spiders. I believe that you do. Let us talk about how we can help you to feel safe."

  Rationale: These approaches provide reality orientation and a sense of safety.

- **Intervention:** Make sure you understand what the patient means. Ask questions and summarize what you think has been said.

  Rationale: Misinterpretation can occur easily.

- **Intervention:** Help patients determine when and why they become anxious. Use problem solving with them to find ways to cope with anxiety. Do this before or after, not during, a psychotic episode.

  Rationale: Anxiety can stimulate signs and symptoms of psychosis.

- **Intervention:** Use physical contact cautiously.

Rationale: Patients who believe they are being persecuted or who are irrational may misinterpret physical contact and overreact.

- **Intervention:** Communicate observations to the physician.

  Rationale: The physician most likely will order an antipsychotic medication to alleviate the signs and symptoms of psychosis.

CASE STUDY

A 47-year-old man was admitted to the hospital 3 weeks ago for evaluation of a possible brain tumor or aneurysm. Before admission, he was markedly healthy. His one sign, which prompted him to seek the care of a physician, was a drooping eyelid. The droop had increased slowly over the course of 1 week, and the lid had closed fully on the 7th day.

After an extensive workup including computed tomography, brain scans, electroencephalography, magnetic resonance imaging, and numerous radiographic studies and hematologic tests, a diagnosis of Burkitt's lymphoma, a rare illness, was made. The patient was scheduled for neurosurgery to implant a shunt that would allow chemotherapeutic agents to be administered directly into his brain.

This patient had no previous history of emotional problems, but throughout the course of his 3-week hospitalization had shown gradually increasing signs of anxiety about the eventual outcome of his illness.

The morning after the neurosurgery, the nurse, Ms. Smith, notices that the patient is markedly agitated. He is gesturing with his arm and seems to be mumbling and whispering. He says to Ms. Smith, "Nurse, nurse, there's a conspiracy going on here. Did you know that? Dr. Jones and Dr. Black are playing with my head; they're doing some kind of mind games. I have been seeing things flying around the room all night. Are these hallucinations or what? Get Dr. Smith; he's the only good one left. I don't trust the rest. Hurry, hurry!" The patient seems to be about to pull out his IV line and jump out of the bed. As he is talking, his agitation is increasing.

Although Ms. Smith is somewhat apprehensive, she does the following:

- With a calm demeanor and using a low modulated voice, introduces herself and reminds the patient where he is and about his recent surgery.

- Assures the patient that she understands his beliefs and believes he is experiencing hallucinations. She tells him that hallucinations are understandable because of his stress over the surgery and severe illness and says that she does not see things flying around the room.

- Indicates to another staff member that she might need some help in restraining this patient for the patient's safety.

- Reports the patient's psychosis and agitation to his physicians.

- Monitors the patient's behaviors often. Stays with him and does an assessment by using a mini–mental status examination.

- Frequently orients the patient and does reality tests.

- Clearly and concisely explains all procedures necessary.

This man's psychosis may have stemmed from a variety of causes:

- His neurosurgery

- His brain disease

- His prolonged hospitalization with the multiple, some invasive, diagnostic procedures

- Some of his medications

Chances are good that this episode will be brief and transient. Most likely, the patient will return to his nonpsychotic state within hours once appropriate treatment is started.

EXAM QUESTIONS

CHAPTER 6
Questions 39–43

39. What does the term psychosis mean?

    a. Smelling things

    b. An inflated belief in oneself

    c. Having hallucinations or delusions or both

    d. A major tranquilizer

40. Altered thought processes is a nursing diagnosis for which of the following?

    a. Cognitive dissonance

    b. Psychiatric dysfunction

    c. Psychosis

    d. Psychoanalysis

41. A person who has a looseness of associations may be which of the following?

    a. Hysterical

    b. Bulimic

    c. Psychotic

    d. Sad

42. What is the definition of echolalia?

    a. Repetition of what someone else says

    b. Repetition of one's own words

    c. A cationic stupor

    d. Psychosis

43. When a nurse is assessing a psychotic patient, it is important to do which of the following?

    a. Check for lethality.

    b. Establish a therapeutic relationship.

    c. Document evidence of psychotic communication.

    d. Get a full medical history.

CHAPTER 7

NURSING MANAGEMENT OF THE CHEMICALLY DEPENDENT PATIENT

CHAPTER OBJECTIVE

After completing this chapter, the reader will be able to recognize chemically dependent and impaired patients and will be able to discuss interventions appropriate in the nursing care of such patients.

LEARNING OBJECTIVES

After studying this chapter, the reader will be able to

1. Specify the DSM-IV alcohol-related diagnoses.

2. Select the theories of causation for alcoholism.

3. Specify the early warning signs of alcoholism.

4. Recognize alcohol-related physical complications.

5. Indicate the signs and symptoms of alcohol withdrawal.

6. Choose the correct psychopharmacologic agents helpful in the treatment of alcohol withdrawal.

7. Indicate which treatments for alcoholism are currently available.

8. Recognize the signs and symptoms of amphetamine abuse.

9. Recognize the signs and symptoms of cocaine overdose and of cocaine withdrawal.

10. Recognize the signs and symptoms of heroin overdose and of heroin withdrawal.

11. Specify the signs and symptoms of abuse of sedatives, hypnotics, and anxiolytics and of withdrawal from these medications.

12. Indicate the theories of causation for drug abuse.

13. Recognize different approaches in the treatment of drug abuse.

OVERVIEW

Nursing management of patients who are chemically dependent on alcohol or drugs or both has become important as the number of such patients has increased. Nurses who work in emergency departments have been familiar with the substance abuser as a patient for a long time. In some parts of the United States, cocaine, crack, and PCP have brought increased violence into the emergency department. Drug-related problems are seen on medical-surgical units and even on the maternity units, where drug-addicted mothers are giving birth to drug-addicted babies. Some of these occurrences are being reported on the nightly news in some of the bigger cities.

ALCOHOLISM

Alcohol is the most pervasive substance of abuse of all chemicals. Alcohol addiction knows no barriers. Men, women, teenagers, the elderly, and even young children have experienced the problems of alcoholism. Numerous medical complications are associated with alcohol abuse, and patients in the general hospital, who are there for any number of reasons, also can be in an early or later stage of alcohol-related disease. Because denial is such a strong component of alcoholism, many alcoholics avoid confrontation.

The bedside nurse may be an alcoholic patient's earliest contact with a health care provider. Thus, the nurse has the first opportunity to intervene by providing assessment, corroboration, referral, and collaboration with the patient and the members of the patient's health team and family. The bedside nurse may make an impact on or at least a dent in the resistance of this patient. Therefore nurses should use good interpersonal techniques and be aware of their own attitude toward chemically dependent patients.

Alcohol is a liquid chemical that acts as a CNS depressant. Although some early signs and symptoms of intoxication, such as giddiness, talkativeness, loosening of inhibitions, and relaxation, seem socially appealing, contrary to popular belief, alcohol is not a stimulant.

Alcohol acts differently in each person. Some of the effects are related to each person's absorption time, which can be affected by variables such as the following:

- Amount of alcohol consumed
- How fast the alcoholic drinks follow each other
- The person's body weight, height, and general size
- Presence or absence of food in the stomach
- Stomach emptying time, metabolic rate
- How much time has passed while the person was drinking

Alcohol abuse is a complex process whereby both a psychological and a physical dependence on alcohol has occurred progressively. Alcoholics are unable to stop drinking and often drink to excess.

A description of alcoholism includes items such as the amount and frequency of alcohol consumption and any evidence of the signs and symptoms of alcohol withdrawal. An assessment should be made of the person's dependence on drinking and of the possible sequelae of social problems, such as marital, work-related, or possible problems with the law (e.g., drunk driving or arrests for fighting). Physical illnesses, such as liver problems and disease, stomach ailments, and neurologic problems, and recurrent trauma can provide clues to alcoholism. Emotional problems, such as depression, insomnia, and irritability, can be indications of alcohol abuse.

Alcoholism is a progressive disease, and it can be fatal. The DSM-IV diagnosis of alcoholism at a pathologic level is alcohol dependence or alcohol abuse. Abuse refers to patterns of alcohol use with the continuation of drinking despite marital discord, job threats, and physical problems. An example of someone who abuses alcohol is a person who continues to drink and drive, seemingly unaware of the danger, despite statistics showing that 50% of all automobile accidents involve drivers who have been drinking. Alcohol dependence is diagnosed on the basis of persistence, craving, and continual use and generally is thought to include a withdrawal syndrome.

The progressive course of alcoholism can range from mild signs and symptoms of hangover, missing or being late to work, and some marital discord to total craving and dependence on alcohol. Alcohol dependence may be associated with a complete breakdown in the family, a loss of job, poor health, and signs and symptoms of withdrawal.

Other DSM-IV diagnoses related to alcoholism include the following:

- Alcohol-induced persisting dementia

- Alcohol-induced persisting amnestic disorder
- Alcohol-induced psychotic disorder, with delusions
- Alcohol-induced psychotic disorder, with hallucinations
- Alcohol-induced mood disorder
- Alcohol-induced anxiety disorder
- Alcohol-induced sexual dysfunction
- Alcohol-induced sleep disorder
- Alcohol intoxication
- Alcohol withdrawal
- Alcohol intoxication delirium
- Alcohol withdrawal delirium

According to a Gallup poll, one in four families is affected adversely by alcohol use or abuse. The alcoholic is affected directly, and the alcoholic's family may be affected emotionally, socially, financially, or medically.

Theories of Causation

At this time, no single definitive cause of alcoholism is known. Nevertheless, many aspects of alcoholism are well known, including common problems and issues for possible causation. Early warning signs and generalities are earmarks of potential problems. A combination of physical, psychological, and social factors seems logical, in the context of each alcoholic's personal life.

Physical factors. Because a high rate of alcoholism is seen in families, a genetic link cannot be ruled out. Another theory is that an endocrine dysfunction may cause a demand or a predisposition for alcohol.

Psychological factors. Psychological factors include extreme dependence, needing "oral" gratification, and drinking for relief of tension.

Social factors. Social factors include excessive drinking as a result of patterns found in the family and being "socialized" to drink at a young age. In addition, some cultural and ethnic groups drink more than others do, and more men than women are alcoholics, although the number of women with alcoholism is increasing.

Other theories. The allergy theory proposes that in some persons the body has an allergic response to alcohol. A nutritional theory claims that some deficiencies may cause a craving for alcohol.

Warning Signs of Alcoholism

The warning signs of alcoholism include the following:

- A loss of control over drinking, sneaking drinks, drinking until unconscious, drinking in the morning
- Social and occupational problems with drinking: Arguing about drinking with spouse and other family members, missing work because of drinking or being hung over, not keeping engagements, becoming unreliable
- Blackout episodes, times when the person is functioning but has no recall for events
- Possible legal complications: Being stopped and ticketed by police for driving under the influence of alcohol

Medical Complications

A number of physiologic problems and potential diseases are related to excessive drinking. *Table 7-1* gives some of the physical complications associated with alcoholism. Patients who have these problems may show up first in the general hospital for treatment of the alcohol-related problem or because of other health-related issues. The presence of these problems may provide clues to a patient's covert alcoholism.

Alcohol Intoxication

People who are intoxicated are usually not too difficult to recognize. They generally have some or all of the following:

- Odor of alcohol on the breath

Table 7-1
Alcohol-Related Physical Complications

System or Organs Involved	Complication
Brain, neurologic	Peripheral polyneuritis
	Wernicke-Korsakoff syndrome (disorientation, delirium, confusion, confabulation, ocular impairment; a progressive disorder that requires thiamine replacement)
Liver, pancreas	Alcoholic hepatitis Liver failure Pancreatitis
Muscle	Myopathy
Cardiopulmonary	Enlarged heart Susceptibility to infections Pneumonia
Gastrointestinal	Gastric distress Ulcers Nutritional imbalance
Hematologic	Anemia

- Emotional lability, euphoria-hostility
- Slurred speech
- Ataxia, incoordination
- Poor judgment
- Decreased inhibitions, aggressiveness, increased sexual impulses
- Memory impairment

Alcohol Withdrawal

In a general hospital, a patient can be a secret alcoholic and be in the hospital for a problem that is related or unrelated to alcoholism. Because patients may have to suddenly cease drinking when they are admitted, nurses must be aware of the signs and symptoms of alcohol withdrawal. These include the following:

- Autonomic hyperactivity
- Tremors, especially of hands and face

- Tachycardia
- Psychomotor agitation
- Anxiety
- Nausea
- Vomiting
- Insomnia
- Seizures
- Transient hallucinations
- Delusions
- Delirium tremens

Withdrawal from alcohol generally occurs 24–72 hr after the last drink was taken. During withdrawal, the patient's health progressively deteriorates. Potential complications of alcohol withdrawal include the following:

- Aspiration pneumonia
- Peripheral vascular collapse

- Hyperthermia

- Infection

- Myocardial infarction

- Self-inflicted trauma, purposeful or accidental

- Death, because of one of the other complications

The immediate treatment of withdrawal for present or impending delirium tremens is pharmacologic. A minor tranquilizer, usually a benzodiazepine such as Librium (chlordiazepoxide) or Ativan (lorazepam), is used. The CNS depressant action of the drug helps minimize progression of the withdrawal. The benzodiazepine then can be titrated down gradually to the lowest effective dose until the patient is no longer at risk for serious sequelae of withdrawal. Eventually the medication can be discontinued.

Other problems to be considered are the patient's nutritional status, including fluid and electrolyte balance and levels of vitamins, thiamine, and magnesium. The potential for trauma or self-harm should be addressed as appropriate. Obviously, any imminent crisis (e.g., circulatory or respiratory collapse) must be attended to immediately.

Treatments for Alcoholism

When the immediate effects of alcohol withdrawal are subsiding, the ongoing treatment for alcoholism as the primary disease problem needs to be considered. Most treatment programs in the United States are based on the idea of the "recovering" alcoholic. These programs advocate taking 1 day at a time, accepting the idea that the temptation to drink is ever-present in our society and that abstinence is the only way to maintain sobriety.

A variety of programs are available. Inpatient programs are found in general hospitals, psychiatric hospitals, residential treatment facilities, and group homes. Outpatient treatment can be privately based or through the auspices of clinics, hospitals, or other public facilities.

Of all of the outpatient programs, Alcoholics Anonymous (AA) is the most well known and widely used of the 12-step programs. It is free, anonymous, and supportive, and since the 1940s has been a growing, well-used, and well-respected self-help program.

Public and private outpatient programs are available through clinics and private practitioners of a variety of disciplines, including physicians, nurses, social workers, psychologists, and drug and alcohol counselors. These programs may be group or individual oriented. Some offer residential treatment and then outpatient follow-up care.

Use of medications beyond withdrawal has been effective. Antabuse (disulfiram) is sometimes used as an alcohol antagonist. Some patients who cannot achieve sobriety independently find taking Antabuse just enough of a deterrent to maintain abstinence. However, the benefits are eliminated if the patient has no motivation for taking the antagonist.

Because the causes of alcoholism differ from person to person, a wide range of treatment approaches are effective. Self-help groups other than AA are available, including family and marital therapy (which can be an important adjunct as well), individual therapy, education programs, behavioral therapy, and aversion therapy.

Each person's situation, general health, emotional problems, amount of alcoholic disease, and life circumstances should be considered when recommendations for treatment are made. It may be preferable for the alcoholic to be an inpatient for a while, removed from the pressures and commitments of everyday life, in a place where treatment can be intensive and last all day. Alternatively, being an inpatient may jeopardize a person's job, family, or social situation, and thus, beginning treatment as an outpatient is a better option.

The trend in treatment is a multisystem effort. Programs include many different approaches.

Usually a patient's treatment plan includes the following:

- Individual counseling

- Group therapy

- Daily educational meeting

- Family therapy

- Occupational therapy or vocational rehabilitation

- Recreational therapy

- Psychopharmacologic therapy

The increasing problem of alcoholism and the increased attention given to it by the medical community and the media have brought the "secret" of widespread abuse of alcohol out in the open. Treatment options are widely available to all who are comfortable in admitting they are alcoholic and in seeking help.

DRUG ABUSE

Drug abuse has always been around. Stories have been told of opium dens, mescaline dreams, and herbs and spirits used for changing the level of consciousness and awareness and for enhancing mood. The drug of choice has varied, depending on the time and the country. At times, some drugs were legal and others were illegal (e.g., cocaine and alcohol).

Aside from alcohol, heroin has long been a substance of abuse. In the 1960s, marijuana, LSD, and other psychedelic drugs were the popular drugs of choice. Simultaneously came the popularity of "downers" (barbiturates and tranquilizers) and the abuse of prescribed medicine. In the 1970s, "uppers" came to the forefront, along with PCP. The 1980s brought the cocaine crisis, including crack, and crystal methamphetamine (crystal meth). All the previous drug problems continued as well.

Epidemic proportions are true for some drugs, and certainly the whole problem of drug abuse is an epidemic crisis. In the 1990s, the issue of drug abuse persists. Use of crack cocaine is particularly dangerous, because its users often turn to violent crimes in order to support their habit.

Is the tide turning? Awareness of drug abuse and education about it are increasing. Grass-roots groups such as Mothers Against Drunk Driving (MADD) started small and have become major organizations, with political clout, to help combat the problems. Nancy Reagan's campaign Just Say No to Drugs helped highlight the problems and needs. The drug program does seem to have a backlash, but it is hoped that the steady increase in drug abuse will be affected by the fight against the problem.

The groups of substances of abuse other than alcohol that are listed in DSM-IV for both substance abuse and dependence include the following:

- Amphetamines

- Caffeine

- Cannabis

- Cocaine

- Hallucinogens

- Inhalants

- Nicotine

- Opioids

- PCP

- Sedatives, hypnotics, anxiolytics

- Polysubstances

Amphetamines

Amphetamines are CNS stimulants. Although no longer widely prescribed, these drugs often were prescribed as diet pills and have a side benefit of being pep pills. They are still used in the medical management of hyperactivity in children and increasingly in the elderly. Research has verified that short-term, low doses of Ritalin (methylphenidate) are effective treatment for depression in the elderly. Amphetamines are generally avoided medically because of their high potential for abuse. The signs and symptoms of amphetamine abuse are as follows:

- Euphoria
- Hyperalertness
- Anorexia
- Increased pulse rate
- Increased blood pressure
- Insomnia
- Excessive talkativeness

Cannabis

Marijuana and hashish generally produce a state of mild euphoria and relaxation. These illegal drugs are smoked in a "joint," a home-rolled cigarette, or through a pipe. Hallucinations can occur with high doses. Lack of motivation and possible irreversible brain damage have been of concern in adolescents who smoke marijuana.

Cocaine

Cocaine seems to have been the scourge of the 1980s. When cocaine abuse first became widespread, it was considered a white-collar problem. The drug was expensive, and initially addiction and withdrawal problems were not seen.

A fast-acting but short-lasting CNS stimulant, cocaine produces a rush of euphoria. The popularity of "coke," as it is commonly known, has continued and spread. The drug has found its way into poorer communities as crack cocaine, a cheaper, less pure, and smokable form of cocaine. Cocaine addiction has increased, and a withdrawal syndrome is now recognized. The signs and symptoms of cocaine overdose include the following:

- Anxiety-panic
- Increased pulse rate
- Increased blood pressure
- Dilated pupils
- Severe perspiration

- Syncope
- Seizures
- Episodes of delusions, paranoia, hallucinations, and mania
- Death, usually as a result of cardiac or respiratory failure

Hallucinogens

The hallucinogens LSD, PCP, and mescaline are drugs that alter the user's sense of reality and consciousness. They cause a distorted sense of energy and excitement, and hallucinations and other perceptual changes may occur. LSD was popularized as "acid" in the hippie era of the 1960s. In the 1970s, PCP or angel dust was more common. Violent side effects are associated with use of PCP. Users can become quite paranoid and delusional and act out impulsively. Personnel in the emergency department often have been assaulted while attempting to administer care to such patients.

Inhalants

Sniffing glue or inhaling other substances such as paint, paint thinner, gasoline, or even white-out (Liquid Paper) is a less common problem than other forms of drug abuse. Children and preteens are more apt than people in other age groups to use inhalants, probably because the substances are cheap and readily available. Inhalants and some other substances are seen as a "cheap high" in this school-age group and may cause not only social and school problems but also respiratory and brain damage.

Opioids

Heroin, methadone, and narcotics such as morphine and Demerol (meperidine) have long been known for their addictive properties and their definite and severe withdrawal patterns. Abused for their euphoric properties, these drugs also produce pain relief, apathy, and impaired judgment. Heroin addicts seem to be seeking release from daily woes. The signs and symptoms of heroin overdose are as follows:

- Decreased respirations
- Pinpoint pupils
- Pale, cool, clammy skin with cyanotic tinge
- Needle tracks (marks) on the arms and legs or in areas of hidden veins
- Cardiac dysrhythmias
- Clouded consciousness, semicomatose states, coma
- Pulmonary edema
- Shock
- Death as a result of respiratory failure or cerebral edema

Sedatives, Hypnotics, and Anxiolytics

Sedatives, hypnotics, and anxiolytics are a group of tranquilizing drugs that cause quiescence and relaxation and a decrease in tension and anxiety. Still prescribed medically and valuable for their beneficial effects, these drugs are highly misused and abused. Tolerance often develops, causing the need for increases in doses and frequency of use. If outright addiction does not occur, habituation and dependence are common. The signs and symptoms of abuse and overdose of these drugs are as follows:

- Craving and tolerance
- Ataxia
- Irritable mood
- Slurred speech
- Sustained nystagmus
- Slowed reactions
- Lethargy
- Impaired judgment
- Confusion
- Disorientation
- Clouded consciousness
- Hypersomnia
- Coma

Definitions of Terms

Because a range of abuse exists, some clarification of terms may be useful:

- *Abuse:* The misuse of chemical substances, alcohol, and drugs, over a prolonged period of time
- *Habit:* The constant wanting and use of a substance in the absence of a physical dependence, although a psychological dependence may be present
- *Tolerance:* A gradual need to increase the dose or frequency of use (or both) of a substance to obtain the same high
- *Dependence:* A continuous craving and preference to use a substance to maintain a state of physical balance or psychological well-being (or both)
- *Addiction:* A continuous need to take a substance to maintain physical functioning; the absence of the substance causes a physiologic withdrawal syndrome

Theories of Causation

Drug abuse is steadily on the rise. Even though some drugs of abuse are illegal and not always as readily available as alcohol, our society has been medically and commercially socialized to "pop" pills: "Have a headache, toothache? Take an aspirin, Tylenol, Motrin." Children are raised in a comfortable-with-pills atmosphere.

Young people often begin abusing substances because of peer pressure. The vulnerable preteen time and adolescence experienced by some lead to drug-taking behaviors to be part of the crowd and to fit in. Some adolescents may be rebelling against their parents, other authority figures, and society itself. Others may be looking for an escape from their perceived problems and feelings of depression. These children are looking for a way out of their present reality.

Although caution seems to be more prevalent now, the 1960s saw many persons "experiencing" a drug and seeking mood- and mind-altered states. Once substances of abuse are tried, different variables seem to come into play, which determine the course of the drug abuse problem. The user's place in society, self-esteem and self concept, age, peers, finances, life-style, other personality characteristics, and other physical and emotional problems intermingle.

Abuse of prescription medicines may start with a defined ailment. However, use can quickly become a convoluted problem, with increasing reliance on some drugs such as pain killers.

In view of the different drugs readily available, it is no surprise that polysubstance abuse (abusing more than one drug at a time) has become a problem. Although all the drugs used are associated with some degree of psychological dependence, some are physically addicting. They cause a craving and tolerance, and discontinuing them causes a great deal of physical discomfort, so much so that the "need" for the drug is heightened. Heroin addiction is an example of this phenomenon.

Like alcoholism, drug addiction seems to have no single known causative factor. It seems to manifest itself in a person who is experiencing a combination of biological, psychological, and social phenomena.

Many researchers are dissatisfied with the inconclusiveness of psychosocial theories of drug dependence and are focusing their attention on biochemical factors related to drug use. Nothing conclusive has been proved yet.

Signs and Symptoms of Withdrawal

Any patient who is addicted to one or more substances and is now in the general hospital is at risk for withdrawal. The bedside nurse should be aware of the signs and symptoms of withdrawal. Those for cocaine withdrawal include the following (American Psychiatric Association, 1994):

- Dysphoric mood
- Vivid, unpleasant dreams
- Fatigue
- Hypersomnia or insomnia
- Psychomotor retardation or agitation
- Increased appetite

The signs and symptoms of withdrawal from opioids are as follows (American Psychiatric Association, 1994):

- Dysphoric mood
- Nausea, vomiting
- Muscle aches
- Lacrimation or rhinorrhea
- Pupillary dilation, piloerection, or sweating
- Diarrhea
- Yawning
- Fever
- Insomnia

The signs and symptoms of withdrawal from sedatives, hypnotics, or anxiolytics are as follows (American Psychiatric Association, 1994):

- Autonomic hyperactivity
- Increased hand tremors
- Insomnia
- Nausea, vomiting
- Transient visual, tactile, or auditory hallucinations
- Psychomotor agitation
- Anxiety
- Grand mal seizures

Available Treatments

Chemically dependent patients generally cannot achieve a drug-free life-style on their own.

Because of the craving, cost, peer-group pressure, and increased need for the sometimes illegal substances, continued abuse can cause serious damage in the user's life. Family, friends, job relationships, the community, and society at large may all be affected adversely.

As with alcoholism, treatment for a drug addiction should be self-motivated. Although outside forces—job, family, money, and health—can contribute to the reasoning, a chemically dependent person needs to want to quit. Along with the desire to become drug-free, help and support from others are very important.

Both inpatient and residential programs are available. For some patients, the need to be away from a drug-taking environment, place, or people is crucial to gaining freedom from a dependency. Others do better by maintaining their usual activities and find outpatient programs a better option.

In conjunction with an addict's general physical condition and state, the drug of abuse itself may be a factor in determining the best type of treatment. Some emergency or acute medical care may be needed, either for an overdose problem or for potential sequelae of withdrawal.

Hospitals; clinics; popular residential treatment facilities such as the Betty Ford Center in California, Synanon, Phoenix House, and DayTop Village; and hundreds of other private facilities offer a wide range of services. Outpatient programs, methadone clinics, and private practitioners also offer many services. These include the following:

- Individual therapy

- Group therapy, supportive and confrontative

- Family and marital counseling

- 12-Step, anonymous groups

- Self-help recovery groups

- Psychopharmacologic therapy: Generally used for detoxification, in emergencies as antago-

nists, and for maintenance therapy (e.g., methadone for heroin)

Treatment should be individualized for each patient. The single predictive criterion for success or failure for all addicts is the level of motivation or lack of it. When motivation is high, a degree of recovery usually can be achieved.

Recovery is not necessarily an all-or-nothing event. It is common for some slips to occur. Therefore, patients must try again and again. Even though an addict may not remain drug-free, repeated failures should not be criticized. An attitude of acceptance and willingness to support an addict's attempts to attain and maintain a drug-free state should be fostered.

Treatment for withdrawal. For some drugs of abuse associated with a physical withdrawal syndrome, psychopharmacologic treatment is available to help patients withdraw safely. Methadone (Dolophine) is used successfully in withdrawal from heroin. Clonidine (Catapres) is under investigation as a drug for withdrawal from opiates. Benzodiazepines (e.g., Librium and Valium) are used sometimes for withdrawal from tranquilizers, cocaine, and amphetamines. Sometimes the drug of abuse is given in titrated-down doses until the drug is no longer necessary.

NURSING ATTITUDES

For both alcoholics and drug abusers, the manner in which a nurse cares for them can be important. Believing addiction is an illness rather than a moral weakness is helpful. It is a good idea for nurses to examine their own attitudes and beliefs about addicts and addiction before working in this field.

NURSING DIAGNOSES

Numerous nursing diagnoses are possible in patients with an addiction problem. Patients generally have more than one of the following:

- Risk for injury
- Risk for violence, self-directed or directed at others
- Ineffective individual coping
- Chronic low self-esteem
- Altered thought processes
- Sensory or perceptual alteration
- Denial, ineffective
- Spiritual distress
- Altered family process: alcoholism

Diagnoses related to the potential physiologic sequelae of chemical dependency include the following:

- Activity intolerance
- Sleep pattern disturbance
- Anxiety
- Diarrhea
- Altered nutrition: less than body requirements
- Self-care deficit
- Sexual dysfunction

NURSING INTERVENTIONS

The following nursing interventions can be used for patients who are chemically dependent on alcohol or drugs:

- **Intervention:** Provide safety for the patient, from trauma and harm.

  Rationale: While under the influence of a substance, patients cannot maintain their own safety needs.

- **Intervention:** Assess and continually monitor the patient for adverse medical sequelae of intoxication or withdrawal.

  Rationale: Some drugs may cause death as a result of cardiac or respiratory failure.

- **Intervention:** Assess and monitor the patient's mental status.

  Rationale: Mental status changes and fluctuates according to ingestion of the substance and the amount ingested.

- **Intervention:** Provide support and establish rapport and a relationship with the patient.

  Rationale: Support and a rapport with health care providers can help encourage freedom from substance abuse and increase the patient's low self-esteem.

- **Intervention:** Encourage verbalization and exploration.

  Rationale: These measures help the patient recognize his or her problem areas.

- **Intervention:** Teach the patient about substance abuse, including the psychological, biological, and social ramifications.

  Rationale: Knowledge about substance abuse will help the patient recognize the potential for increasing problems.

- **Intervention:** Assess available support and explore options.

  Rationale: Knowledge about available support and possible options can help patients recognize their potential strengths.

- **Intervention:** Provide role modeling.

  Rationale: Role modeling sets an example and shows patients that they can be drug-free.

- **Intervention:** Administer psychopharmacologic medications when necessary as directed by a physician.

- **Intervention:** Encourage the use of and teach relaxation techniques.

  Rationale: Relaxation can provide relief from tension and decrease anxiety.

EXAM QUESTIONS

CHAPTER 7
Questions 44–56

44. Drinking alcohol in the morning on a regular basis is considered which of the following?

    a. Social

    b. An early warning sign of alcoholism

    c. Healthy by some physicians

    d. Helpful for tension relief

45. Seizures, anxiety, and paranoia are signs and symptoms of which of the following?

    a. Psychotic depression

    b. Cocaine overdose

    c. Alcohol intoxication

    d. Dementia

46. Which of the following is characterized by dysphoric mood; vivid, unpleasant dreams; and an increase in appetite?

    a. Heroin use

    b. Suicidal ideation

    c. Cocaine withdrawal

    d. Anorexia nervosa

47. Which of the following are signs or symptoms of amphetamine abuse?

    a. Increased body temperature, increased blood pressure, increased pulse rate

    b. Increased pulse rate, decreased blood pressure, increased temperature

    c. Euphoria, anorexia, increased pulse rate

    d. Anorexia, increased blood pressure, increased body temperature

48. Signs and symptoms of alcohol withdrawal include which of the following?

    a. Delirium tremens, anorexia, headache

    b. Fever, poor judgment, hypersomnia

    c. Tremors, tachycardia, insomnia

    d. Psychosomatic ills, tremors, bradycardia

49. Potential complications of alcohol withdrawal include which of the following?

    a. Pulmonary edema and infection

    b. Anemia and ulcers

    c. Grand mal seizures and myopathy

    d. Aspiration pneumonia and myocardial infarction

50. What are the two commonly used medications for alcohol withdrawal?

    a. Chlordiazepoxide and pentobarbital

    b. Diazepam and triazolam

    c. Chlordiazepoxide and lorazepam

    d. Alcohol and phenobarbital

51. What is the most popular program for supportive treatment of patients with alcoholism?

    a. Aversion therapy

    b. ACA

    c. Family therapy

    d. AA

52. Yawning may be a sign of which of the following?

    a. Alcohol withdrawal

    b. Sedative overdose

    c. Opioid withdrawal

    d. Cocaine withdrawal

53. Which of the following are signs and symptoms of withdrawal from sedatives, hypnotics, and anxiolytics?

    a. Muscle aches, rhinorrhea, yawning

    b. Autonomic hyperactivity, insomnia, anxiety

    c. Fatigue, dysphoric mood, yawning

    d. Insomnia, rhinorrhea, increased appetite

54. The signs and symptoms of heroin overdose include which of the following?

    a. Decreased respirations, pinpoint pupils, pulmonary edema

    b. Depression, fatigue, pinpoint pupils

    c. Shock, increased blood pressure, insomnia

    d. Pinpoint pupils, decreased respiration, mouth sores

55. Peer pressure seems to contribute to which of the following psychiatric problems?

    a. Drug abuse among some teenagers

    b. Early schizophrenic breakdown

    c. Withdrawal

    d. The binge-purge cycle

56. Residential treatment facilities such as Synanon are used for patients who have which of the following problems or disorders?

    a. Depression

    b. Drug abuse problems

    c. Borderline personality disorders

    d. Organic brain syndromes

CHAPTER 8

NURSING MANAGEMENT OF THE CONFUSED PATIENT

CHAPTER OBJECTIVE

At the completing this chapter, the reader will be able to recognize the signs and symptoms of confusion in a patient and be able to apply sound principles of nursing care to confused patients.

LEARNING OBJECTIVES

After studying this chapter, the reader will be able to

1. Recognize the DSM-IV diagnoses related to confusional states.

2. Differentiate between delirium and dementia.

3. Specify predisposing factors for confusion in a patient.

4. Specify three manifestations of Alzheimer's disease.

5. Indicate the characteristics of a confused patient.

6. Indicate the special considerations needed when caring for the elderly.

7. Recognize the nursing diagnoses related to caring for the confused patient.

8. Select nursing interventions that are helpful for the confused patient.

OVERVIEW

Patients who are confused pose special problems for the bedside nurse. Whatever the causative factors, a confused, possibly brain-injured or brain-impaired, patient is not thinking clearly and may misunderstand others as well as be misunderstood. If the confusion is associated with a problem caused by aging, special concerns and care may need to be considered.

Patients with clouded consciousness, memory difficulties, and problems maintaining a reality base may behave bizarrely and not attend to basic functional needs. This condition may snowball and further impair the patient by adding an affective problem, such as depression, that may contribute to an already increasing confusion.

DSM-IV DIAGNOSES

In the past, different sources from medicine, neurology, psychiatry, and nursing have been inconsistent in their definitions of terms related to confusion, clouded consciousness, and impaired cognition. Many of the discrepancies were based on primary diagnoses, causative factors, or functional descriptions. DSM-IV lists the following diagnoses as related to confusional states:

• Delirium due to…(indicate the general medical condition)

• Substance intoxication delirium

- Substance withdrawal delirium

- Delirium due to multiple etiologies

- Delirium not otherwise specified

- Dementia of the Alzheimer's type, with early onset

    Uncomplicated

    With delirium

    With delusions

    With depressed mood

- Dementia of the Alzheimer's type, with late onset

    Uncomplicated

    With delirium

    With delusions

    With depressed mood

- Vascular dementia

    Uncomplicated

    With delirium

    With delusions

    With depressed mood

- Dementia due to HIV disease

- Dementia due to head trauma

- Dementia due to Parkinson's disease

- Dementia due to Huntington's disease

- Dementia due to Pick's disease

- Dementia due to Creutzfeldt-Jakob disease

- Dementia due to…(indicate the general medical condition not listed in the preceding)

- Substance-induced persisting dementia

- Dementia due to multiple etiologies

- Dementia not otherwise specified

DEFINITION OF TERMS

Generally, medical terms such as *organic brain syndrome, organic mental syndrome,* and *organic mental disorder* are seen in textbooks and in patients' medical records. The terms *organic brain syndrome* and *organic brain disorder* may be used to specify brain dysfunctions, perhaps injury associated with trauma or illnesses that directly affect the brain, although these are terms not diagnoses.

Delirium and *dementia* are commonly used terms. They are sometimes misidentified and confused with each other. A delirium generally has an acute onset, is reversible, and lasts a short time. It is characterized by the waxing and waning of consciousness, which does not happen in dementia. Often delirium has a known precipitating event such as trauma, use of toxic substances, or a physical illness. A dementia is usually more insidious. It may be chronic, slowly progressing over time and with aging, perhaps becoming a permanent impairment. The specific cause may or may not be known or fully understood. However, dementia can be caused by an acute event such as a brain infarct.

RELATED PROBLEMS AND PREDISPOSING FACTORS

Associated problems and predisposing factors of confusion include the following:

- Metabolic, endocrine, and electrolyte disturbances

- Respiratory distress, hypoxia

- Chronic liver and kidney disorders

- Neurologic disorders, epilepsy, Parkinson's disease, and CNS infections (e.g., meningitis, encephalitis, syphilis)

- Cancers, tumors

- Cerebrovascular disease

- Systemic infections (e.g., AIDS)

- Nutritional imbalances, vitamin and mineral poisoning or deficiency

- Injury, trauma, embolism

- Toxic effects: substance abuse, alcohol abuse, adverse reactions to medications

- Sensory overload, sensory deprivation, perceptual problems

- Genetic and birth defects, Down syndrome, Huntington's chorea, multiple sclerosis

- Depression

ALZHEIMER'S DISEASE

When we think of a chronic dementia in aging or one known to have a presenile onset, Alzheimer's disease comes to mind. Since the mid-1980s, this disease has been highly publicized and somewhat better understood. The disease begins with sporadic losses of memory and forgetfulness, and impairment becomes greater over time. Mood fluctuations, sometimes inappropriate; perhaps some paranoia; disorientation; speech impairments; and motor impairments all contribute adversely to the person's conscious awareness and cognitive thinking. Nursing care of patients who have Alzheimer's disease must be concerned with communication patterns and with the effects confusion may have on the patients' safety.

CHARACTERISTICS OF CONFUSION

Because of differences in patients' personality structure and the variety of possible causative factors, each patient's confusion is unique in some manifestations. The general picture of the patient who is confused may be as follows:

- The patient may have difficulty remembering recent events before or during the hospitalization. Patients may not remember what they are being told about their condition or care. They may not remember instructions given to them. In addition, past memory may be effected.

- The patient may deny that any problems exist and confabulate, becoming quite agitated when confronted with this behavior.

- The patient may be disoriented about time, place, and possibly person. Patients may misidentify day with night, day of the week, or date of the month and year. They may not know where they are; this state may fluctuate—sometimes they are accurate, sometimes not. In situations of severe disorientation, patients may not know who they are, although this condition is rare. More commonly, patients do not know who you are and need reminding of your name and role at each interaction.

- Disorientation usually becomes more severe as evening comes, a condition referred to as *sundowning*. With decreases in light and stimulation at night, the patient is less able to distinguish between stimuli. Increased agitation can be associated with sundowning.

- The patient may have impaired thought processes. Patients may show a lack of good judgment, be apathetic, show evidence of illogical thinking, seem deficient in their fund of general knowledge, and be unable to perform simple mathematical calculations.

- The patient may be suspicious, paranoid, scared, frightened, and out of touch with reality.

- The patient's speaking may be affected and sometimes may become strange and bizarre. Motor coordination and the ability to walk or lift may be impaired. Facial expressions and changes in affect may be inappropriate.

- The patient may be regressed behaviorally, experience loss of control over bodily functions such as bladder or bowel functions, or have a specific body part affected because of brain damage. Some patients may be incapable of performing basic activities of daily living and need complete care and monitoring.

- Patients may express themselves inappropriately sexually, perhaps disrobing compulsively or masturbating publicly.

The potential reversibility of some or all of these problems depends on the causative factor. An acute delirium caused by drugs or alcohol should dissipate with time and detoxification. A more chronic problem such as cardiovascular problems or Alzheimer's disease will result in continuous deficits of various degrees.

CARING FOR THE ELDERLY

Although confusion has many reasons and occurs in persons of all ages, its prevalence is higher among the elderly. Aging is a natural process of change in all body organs and potential functioning that may lead to deficits in cognition. Older persons have more potential for disease, whether because an illness manifests itself in later life or because a body that is older and has a more diminished capacity is subject to potential ill health. Whichever, the elderly often are at risk for confusion.

The *graying of America,* a term coined for the increase in the number of persons who are more than 65 years old, has had an impact on health care. The longer humans live, the more diseases and health problems they have. The elasticity and flexibility of the body also are decreased in older patients, and it may take them longer to get well or even partially recover their health. For some, if it is not one medical crisis, it is another, perhaps two or three at a time.

Nevertheless, each patient is an individual. An elderly person who is confused should not be writ-

ten off as senile and incapable of understanding or improving communication. As with all confusion, a careful assessment should be made to determine any potentially reversible causes.

Some elderly persons are prone to depression, possibly reactive depression associated with grieving for losses that combines with other factors to culminate in a full-blown depression. Depression in the elderly may appear to be or manifest itself as a pseudodementia. Once the depression is treated and lifted, the dementia should dissipate also.

Older people may have physical changes that cause increased susceptibility to the potency or toxic effects of certain medications. Even medications a person has been taking for a long time can pose new problems because of bodily changes. Some confused elderly persons may wander and be a danger to themselves if they are lost. Bone changes may pose another danger of potential injury. Visual and hearing acuity may lessen, posing another potential threat to high-level functioning.

The elderly may succumb to certain psychiatric disorders. Treatment regimens are generally the same for any age group. However, because of the potential side effects, treatment with some psychopharmacologic agents may be unsuccessful in the elderly. A treatment such as ECT (for depression) may be safer.

Issues of safety, especially the potential need for and use of mechanical restraints, must be considered carefully. Patients must be monitored to avoid injury caused by the restraints themselves, by fighting against them, or as a result of sequelae of stasis.

Elderly patients justly deserve the optimum of nursing care, delivered with thoughtful consideration for maintaining the patients' dignity.

NURSING DIAGNOSES

Nursing diagnoses for patients who have confusion may include the following:

- Altered thought processes

- Sensory or perceptual alteration

- Risk for injury

- Risk for violence, self-directed or directed at others

- Self-esteem disturbance

- Anxiety

- Impaired memory

NURSING INTERVENTIONS

The following nursing interventions can be used for patients who have confusion:

- **Intervention:** Assess the level of confusion or disorientation by doing a mental status examination.

  Rationale: The amount of confusion and its possible cause will help determine the patient's needs and abilities.

- **Intervention:** Do reality testing with the patient.

  Rationale: Monitoring the fluctuations in the patient's level of awareness and comprehension enables you to make necessary changes in the care plan.

- **Intervention:** Reorient the patient: Use calendars, a clock, the newspaper, radio, television, your person; make frequent visits.

  Rationale: Helping patients maintain a reality base can decrease deficits from memory impairment and increase the patients' ability to feel safe and aware.

- **Intervention:** Provide an environment that keeps the patient safe from injury and potential self-harm.

Rationale: A safe environment decreases the potential for trauma and accidents.

- **Intervention:** Decrease environmental stimuli.

  Rationale: Increases in stimuli can increase patients' anxiety, which can compound their inability to comprehend correctly.

- **Intervention:** Use simple communications, simple words, short sentences; be frequently repetitious.

  Rationale: Clear communications can increase patients' ability to comprehend, remember, and follow directions.

- **Intervention:** Devise memory assistance tools: the patient's name on the door, large signs for bathroom and room number, big-print calendar, signs in the hallway to the dining room and nursing station, and so forth.

  Rationale: Helping patients remember and maintain orientation increases their independence.

- **Intervention:** Administer psychotropic medications as ordered, but judiciously.

  Rationale: Decreasing anxiety, psychosis, and depression can relieve patients' confusion or level of confusion and comprehension. Judicious administration is called for because these medications can increase the confusion and add or increase a delirium.

- **Intervention:** Use soft restraints when necessary, and check them often.

  Rationale: Restraints may be the last safety measure for patients who wander and are potentially dangerous to their own health or have a serious and imminent potential for assaultiveness.

- **Intervention:** Offer support and provide reassurance.

  Rationale: Support and reassurance can increase patients' trust in you and give them a feeling of safety and security.

- **Intervention:** Treat confused patients with dignity and respect. Use their proper names; do not treat them as if they were children.

  Rationale: Being treated with dignity and respect increases patients' self-esteem and self-concept.

- **Intervention:** Encourage independence in choices and functioning.

  Rationale: Making choices and functioning independently can increase patients' feelings of self-worth and improve their ability to rely on themselves.

- **Intervention:** Give positive feedback for correct responses and appropriate independent behaviors.

  Rationale: Positive feedback can reinforce appropriate behavior and increase patients' feelings of self-esteem.

- **Intervention:** Provide the patient's family with information on confusion and its underlying causes and treatment.

  Rationale: The patient's family may be worried or angry because of the patient's confusion.

CASE STUDY

Mrs. Gold, a 69-year-old woman, was admitted to a medical unit with a diagnosis of pneumonia of the left lung. Mr. Gold, the patient's husband, was out of town on an extended business trip when the couple's daughter-in-law, Joan Dolan, noted that Mrs. Gold was quite fatigued, breathless at times, and complaining of chest pain. Joan brought Mrs. Gold to a hospital emergency room because Mrs. Gold did not have a regular physician and apparently had not had a checkup in many years.

Mrs. Gold was admitted to her room at 4:30 p.m., and after a few minutes visiting, Joan left her mother-in-law and went home. Jim Vincent was Mrs. Gold's primary nurse for the evening shift, and he went to her room at 5 p.m. to do an initial assessment. Mrs. Gold was not in her room; she was found standing in front of a patient's room two doors down the hallway. Jim escorted Mrs. Gold back to her room and did a nursing assessment.

The assessment included a mini mental status examination, which Jim thought the patient had a great deal of difficulty answering. He decided to do a more complete mental status examination and was continually concerned with Mrs. Gold's level of confusion.

Jim then accurately intervened as follows:

- Oriented Mrs. Gold to the unit and to her room.

- Labeled Mrs. Gold's room number with her name.

- Oriented Mrs. Gold to time, place, and person.

- Wrote down his own name and the telephone number of Mrs. Gold's daughter-in-law, which he got from the chart, on a piece of paper and taped the paper to Mrs. Gold's bedside stand.

- Notified the physician of his findings and concerns.

- Charted the findings of the mental status examination.

- Alerted the other staff members to Mrs. Gold's confusion problem.

- Checked on Mrs. Gold every 15–30 min, assessing her and orienting her as needed.

The reason for Mrs. Gold's confusion was not immediately apparent or determined. There were no old records to document her mental state. No physician knew her, her husband was out of town, and her daughter-in-law was already in transit. In time, with a thorough workup done for this problem, a cause and perhaps a cure would be found. Nevertheless, in the interim, Mrs. Gold's safety needed to be monitored.

Despite the precipitant for the confusion, nursing interventions could be implemented from the outset. The staff of general hospital units need to be knowledgeable about the problem of confusion and the management of confused patients.

EXAM QUESTIONS

CHAPTER 8
Questions 57–62

57. A metabolic disturbance, substance abuse, and brain injury are all problems that can precipitate which of the following psychiatric conditions?

    a. Schizophrenia

    b. Confusion

    c. Schizoaffective illness

    d. Alzheimer's disease

58. Which of the following are nursing interventions for managing a confused patient?

    a. Do a reality test, monitor vital signs, and reorient the patient.

    b. Assess nutritional status, do a reality test, and provide for the patient's safety.

    c. Do a reality test, reorient the patient, and provide for the patient's safety.

    d. Monitor vital signs, provide support and reassurance, and assess nutritional status.

59. Which of the following are three manifestations of Alzheimer's disease?

    a. Loss of memory, mood fluctuations, speech impairment

    b. Loss of memory, loss of sleep, loss of self-esteem

    c. Mood swings, mental illness, anorexia

    d. Loss of memory, mood swings, bulimia

60. Disorientation to time, place, and person is an indication of which of the following psychiatric conditions?

    a. Schizophrenia

    b. Confusion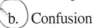

    c. Catatonic excitement

    d. Bipolar affective illness

61. Which of the following considerations should be given priority in the management of a confused 86-year-old woman?

    a. Hygiene

    b. Hearing

    c. Safety

    d. Privacy

62. Pseudodementias are often a manifestation of depression in which age group?

    a. Children

    b. Adolescents

    c. Adults

    d. The elderly

CHAPTER 9

NURSING MANAGEMENT OF THE PATIENT WITH AN EATING DISORDER

CHAPTER OBJECTIVE

After completing this chapter, the reader will be able to recognize the manifestations of the eating disorders anorexia nervosa and bulimia nervosa.

LEARNING OBJECTIVES

After studying this chapter, the reader will be able to

1. Specify the theories of causation for eating disorders.

2. Recognize the signs and symptoms of anorexia nervosa.

3. Specify the manifestations of anorexia nervosa.

4. Specify two signs and symptoms of bulimia nervosa.

5. Indicate the key element in diagnosing bulimia nervosa.

6. Recognize the manifestations of bulimia nervosa.

7. Indicate different treatment options for eating disorders.

8. Indicate the nursing diagnoses that can apply to patients who have eating disorders.

9. Recognize which nursing interventions are helpful when working with a patient who is anorectic or bulimic.

Anorexia nervosa and bulimia nervosa are two psychobiological eating disorders that have grown to epidemic proportions. In January 1989, the California State Assembly resolved to declare an Eating Disorders Week to inform the public of the risks and dangers of this problem. The statistics cited at this Assembly included the estimations that 1 of 200 teenagers 12–18 years old has anorexia nervosa and that 7 million females and 1 million males are affected.

Anorexia nervosa, the oldest, better known of the two disorders, may include self-starvation to the point of emaciation because of a distorted self-image of being fat. Some evidence in medical history fosters a psychosocial belief that women have attempted for many years to gain some mastery over men or control over their own lives and destinies through self-starvation. In those times when women were suppressed, when they had little or no independence or power, the ability to control one's weight and health may have been seen as a powerful tool. How many of us remember the scene in *Gone with the Wind* in which Scarlett O'Hara and her mammy have a power struggle over what to eat and when? This type of power struggle has been played out for various reasons many times.

Historically anorexia nervosa was reported only occasionally. However, in the United States, since the 1970s, this disorder and, as an offshoot, bulimia have become almost common problems. In 1985, the third revised edition of the *Diagnostic and Statistical Manual of Mental Disorders* included bulimia as a separate disease with its own definitions and treatment considerations. The binge-purge cycle previously considered part of the syndrome of anorexia nervosa now is seen regularly in young women on college campuses. Some think anorexia and bulimia are two parts of a continuous disease process that have some similar and some different signs and symptoms. The severity and danger of these signs and symptoms vary from person to person.

Society contributes to the occurrence of these disorders by fostering a goal of what young women ought to look like. Currently it is popular to be thin as well as body conscious. This socialization and acceptance of a norm have helped hide the dangers of these diseases.

Patients who have anorexia nervosa may be seen on general hospital units when they have become so thin that their lives may be in jeopardy, and medical interventions, along with or independent of psychiatric treatment, are necessary to sustain life. Patients who have bulimia generally maintain their weight at a level that is close to average or slightly less than normal weight. Generally the risk of death is small.

A third eating disorder, not talked about as much, is obesity. Although dieting may be on everyone's mind, morbid obesity as a medical and psychiatric disorder is not treated as commonly as anorexia or bulimia. Patients who are morbidly obese may be seen on general hospital units specifically because of their weight problem or because of other health problems. Obesity leads to many health-related illnesses; cardiac, circulatory, and respiratory disorders are potentially fatal problems.

THEORIES OF CAUSATION

The eating disorders have no known causes, despite commonalties from patient to patient. Some acknowledged beliefs for causative factors exist, and, as in other areas of psychiatry, research in this area is ongoing.

One theory proposes developmental crises as the cause. Perhaps some block or stoppage in a child's developmental level during the oral stage of growth leaves the child dependent, unable to separate appropriately and unable to succeed. Adolescence may be another stage for a possible developmental crisis. Because so many patients with anorexia begin to have signs and symptoms during their early teens, it seems possible that the disease is a pathologic development of an adolescent in turmoil. Self-concept, identity, and body image are so important during adolescence.

Another possible psychological cause or interpretation of self-starvation is that the self-gratification and pleasure attached to eating are equated with selfishness and evil. Controlling the natural drive to eat symbolically represents the struggle of the will with more base needs and desires.

Anorexia can also represent a rejection of one's own sexuality or be a punishment for real or imagined transgressions. Nearly starving oneself to death can be a severe denial of the self and the right to exist.

Sociologic theories look at the control factor. Perhaps anorexia is an attempt to exert control over parents. Family treatment often is included as part of a total treatment regimen. The environmental influence of the media on thinness may be a factor. In some cultures, ours being one, thinness is highly desired and is a contributing factor. With the increase in the prevalence of anorexia nervosa, a peer-support theory needs to be considered as well.

Physiologic theories include the possibility of a neuroendocrine abnormality in the area of the hypothalamus that may contribute to a dysfunction in the satiety center of the brain. The exact linkage is not clear. Most likely, a combination of events determines what causes eating disorders and to what extent.

SIGNS AND SYMPTOMS

Anorexia Nervosa

Although anorexia and bulimia nervosa have many signs and symptoms, with some overlapping and some differences in intensity, the following criteria are generally included as necessary for the diagnosis of anorexia nervosa:

- A disturbance in body image

- An intense fear of gaining weight that is not relieved after weight loss occurs

- A body weight of 85% or less of the expected norm

- An absence of menses in postmenarcheal females

The disorder manifests itself in the following ways:

- A refusal to eat anything or anything of substance

- A severe weight loss with emaciation often described as a waiflike appearance or looking like a "concentration camp victim"

- A preoccupation with food, reading food magazines, cooking elaborate meals for others but not eating any of the food prepared

- Strange and bizarre food habits, (e.g., stealing and hoarding food, though not eating it, or setting places at the table in a specific and compulsive manner)

- Hyperactivity and excessive exercising

- Abuse of diuretics and laxatives

- Chronic constipation

- Skin changes: a yellow tinge or the appearance of lanugo, a fine downy hair; hyperkeratosis

- Loss of hair or changes in its texture (e.g., brittle and dry)

- Hypothermia and bradycardia

- Hypotension

- Leukopenia

- Anemia

- Hypoglycemia

- Hypoproteinemia

- Increased basal metabolic rate

- Malnutrition

- Dehydration

- Electrolyte disturbances

- Normal thyroid function

- Normal adrenal cortical function

Emotionally, patients who are anorectic often are depressed and anxious. Sometimes they are psychotic, and sometimes they have obsessive-compulsive traits. Some have committed suicide, and all anorectic patients should be evaluated for this potential.

Bulimia Nervosa

A person who has bulimia gorges on food repetitively and uncontrollably in a short time; this is the binge. The binge ends with purging or self-induced vomiting, usually accomplished by sticking a finger down the throat. When this is done repetitively, over a long time, a reflexive, uncontrollable pattern of vomiting may develop. Other characteristics of ending the binge include the following:

- Falling asleep

- Being caught while purging

- Being found hiding and gorging

- Having stomachaches and stomach pains

Caloric intake during a binge is high. Foods usually favored are high in sugar and fat.

Although the binge-purge cycle is the key element in bulimia, other characteristic signs and symptoms include the following:

- Chronic dieting with weight fluctuations

- A problem with body-image, usually with distortion and some obsessive concerns

- Stomachaches, potential ulcers, and other chronic gastrointestinal disorders

- Frequent sore throats

- Dental problems (with extensive purging, the calcium of the teeth is worn away by the stomach acid)

- Rectal bleeding

- Malnutrition, electrolyte imbalances, and vitamin deficiencies

TREATMENT OPTIONS

Treatment options for the eating disorders differ according to the severity of the illness and the potential danger from adverse sequelae for which the patient is at risk. For a severely disturbed patient, one who is critically ill because of starvation, medical intervention may be needed first. Long-term treatment for patients with eating disorders is psychiatric therapy.

Although no one type of therapy seems particularly more successful than another, a combination of therapies, for a relatively long time, years perhaps, seems to be somewhat successful. Therapy also seems to be more successful in patients who begin treatment early, soon after the disorder becomes apparent. Therapies that may be included in the treatment regimen include the following:

- Individual psychotherapy

- Group therapy

- Family therapy

- Behavior modification

- Cognitive therapy

- Relaxation techniques

- Hypnosis

- Education

- Occupational therapy

- Recreational therapy

- Nutritional counseling

Psychopharmacologic therapy generally is not thought to be the best treatment method. However, patients may be taking antidepressants, tranquilizers, antipsychotics, or anxiolytics. Periactin (cyproheptadine) has been used as an appetite stimulant. Vitamin supplements may be given adjunctively. In an emergency medical situation, forced feeding may be used. This treatment is usually under the aegis of an inpatient service.

Depending on the level of care needed when the patient seeks treatment, many therapists are available on an inpatient or an outpatient basis. Both types of therapy may be necessary, and one or more inpatient stays may be needed during a long course of illness.

Several eating disorder programs are available. These generally offer inpatient stays as well as outpatient follow-up treatment. Some clinics or residences are attached to hospitals, others are free-standing institutions. Many programs are connected to a wide variety of services and treatment for other problems, such as chemical dependency. Some programs are exclusively for eating disorders.

In a general hospital, on a medical unit, nurses may be caring for patients with eating disorders in the capacity of administering basic and supplemental nutrition. The preferred method is for the patient to eat a balanced and nutritionally complete diet. The nurse can confer with the dietician who will be in charge of this regimen. Additionally, a feeding tube may be necessary to provide supplements to regular meals. These feedings generally are administered by the nursing staff.

Patients, particularly those who already have a distorted body image, dislike being fed through a tube. Some may try to pull it out, may fight against it, or may have behavioral problems during feeding administrations. The nurse can help by being supportive and reassuring and clarifying that the feedings are required for life support, that they are not a punishment.

Patients who are critically ill and in need of great amounts of nutrients or whose gastrointestinal systems cannot tolerate a regular diet or tube feedings may need parenteral nutrition administered through a large vein, such as the subclavian vein. Some patients who need long-term parenteral therapy may have a catheter such as a Hickman catheter implanted surgically into the right atrium. These forms of nutritional support, which may seem extreme, generally are used only in severe situations.

NURSING DIAGNOSES

Nursing diagnoses that may be considered for patients with eating disorders include the following:

- Body image disturbance
- Ineffective individual coping
- Anxiety
- Altered nutrition: less than body requirements
- Ineffective denial
- Fatigue
- Altered thought processes

NURSING INTERVENTIONS

The following nursing interventions can be used with a patient who has an eating disorder:

- **Intervention:** Assess the patient's nutritional status, intake and output, and weight.

  Rationale: In patients with an eating disorder, reaching and maintaining an optimal level of health and well-being may be determined by the patients' nutritional status.

- **Intervention:** Provide one-to-one supervision during meals, and observe the patient closely for any indication of hiding food. Give the patient 30 min to eat and do not encourage him or her to eat during this time.

  Rationale: Patients with an eating disorder are ambivalent about food. They may take a long time to eat and may attempt to hide food to avoid eating or to gorge with later.

- **Intervention:** Observe vital signs, especially in patients who may be at critically low weights.

  Rationale: Eating disorders can be fatal diseases.

- **Intervention:** Assess the patient's mental status.

  Rationale: The patient's mental status gives a baseline reference and helps in monitoring potential changes.

- **Intervention:** Observe for signs and symptoms of anxiety, depression, and psychosis.

  Rationale: Anxiety, depression, and psychosis are common in patients who have eating disorders.

- **Intervention:** Observe for suicidal ideation.

  Rationale: Patients who have eating disorders, particularly anorexia nervosa, may become suicidal.

- **Intervention:** Establish a therapeutic relationship and a positive rapport with the patient.

  Rationale: The patient can benefit from the nurse's use of self as a therapeutic tool.

- **Intervention:** Encourage patients to verbalize their feelings.

  Rationale: Verbalization of feelings can reduce stress and clarify problems.

- **Intervention:** Allow ventilation of feelings of anger.

  Rationale: Some patients experience a

great deal of anger and suppress it; this anger needs to be released in an appropriate manner.

- **Intervention:** Collaborate with other health care providers, such as physicians, social service workers, and dieticians.

  Rationale: Collaboration with other health care providers is necessary to establish and use a working treatment plan.

- **Intervention:** Administer supplemental feedings and medications as ordered.

  Rationale: Supplemental feedings and medication help the patient achieve a satisfactory nutritional status.

- **Intervention:** Provide support and reassurance.

  Rationale: Patients may feel out of control.

- **Intervention:** Observe for potential sabotage of the treatment plan.

  Rationale: Fears of gaining weight and the existence of long-standing habits may cause some patients to sabotage their treatment. Patients with eating disorders may induce vomiting, use laxatives, and throw away food while hospitalized.

CASE STUDY

A 20-year-old woman was admitted to a medical unit of a general hospital for treatment of malnutrition. She weighed 74 lb (33.6 kg) and was 5 ft (1.5 m) tall. She denied being anorectic and claimed to have a problem of low energy—"a definite no-no for an aspiring ballerina," she would say.

Vita Stevens, the patient's primary nurse, correctly believed that the patient had anorexia nervosa and was denying the problem. When Ms. Stevens discussed her concerns with the patient's doctor, he confirmed her suspicions, adding, "I recommended psychiatric consultation but she

refused. She would only agree to come to the hospital for a 'rest and overhaul,' as she put it. I was concerned about her and thought she should come in anyway."

The hospital had a clinical nurse specialist in psychiatric and mental health nursing, Roberta Black, on the staff with whom Ms. Stevens previously had collaborated. Ms. Stevens called her and discussed the nursing care for this patient. A nursing staff meeting was scheduled for a few days later. In the meanwhile, Ms. Black visited the patient and remained in contact with Ms. Stevens.

Later in the week, at the nursing conference, the following information was shared:

The patient appeared much younger than her stated age of 20 years. She had long, straight, brown hair, which lacked luster and was stringy and sparse. She appeared waiflike, with wide eyes and a hollow, gaunt face. Her facies seemed sad. She appeared anxious and paced around the unit a lot, dragging a portable IV pole behind her. The pole carried a bag with a catheter connected to a nasogastric feeding tube.

The nurses who knew the patient agreed that she seemed "strange." She talked incessantly about food but ate less than a small amount. She was very much aware of the nasogastric tube, and at meal times, she was withdrawn and preoccupied; sometimes she would have her eyes closed and she would be muttering. Ms. Stevens thought that the patient was hallucinating at times, because she had noticed the patient gesturing and muttering in a peculiar manner.

Ms. Black was concerned with the patient's denial of the eating disorder. The patient had many of the distressing signs and symptoms of anorexia nervosa. Her behavior was cause for concern. She had been seen taking laxatives surreptitiously, throwing some food away from her regular meal tray, attempting to exercise by doing sit-ups and push-ups, and even attempting a cartwheel when she was temporarily free of tubes and monitors. Additionally, some of the nursing staff thought they had heard her vomiting in the bathroom.

A general medical unit usually is not prepared to provide the wide range of therapeutic options for a patient who has an eating disorder. It was recommended at the nursing conference that the following occur:

- Ms. Black, clinical nurse specialist: Confer with the patient's primary physician about obtaining a psychiatric evaluation.

- Ms. Stevens, primary nurse: Establish a positive therapeutic relationship with the patient. Discuss the signs and symptoms of the patient's illness. Educate the patient about anorexia nervosa. Agree on goals for this hospitalization.

- General nursing staff: Observe the patient's behavior and mood. Evaluate her via a mental status examination. Measure the patient's intake and output and weigh her daily. Observe the patient during mealtimes without encouraging her to eat. Give her 30 min to eat and then remove the tray. Administer feedings via a nasogastric tube as ordered. Maintain open channels of communication; include the patient, her physician, her family, the clinical nurse specialist, and the dietician. Document all interventions carefully and clearly. Also document the patient's mental status, medical status, nutritional requirements, vital signs, and intake and output. Be consistent in approach while following the patient's care plan. Have a conference again as needed.

EXAM QUESTIONS

CHAPTER 9
Questions 63–68

63. An adolescent developmental crisis is a theoretical cause of which of the following problems?
    a. Anorexia nervosa
    b. Schizophrenia
    c. Schizoaffective disorder
    d. Personality disorder

64. The signs and symptoms of anorexia nervosa include which of the following?
    a. A physical illness, fear of obesity, and a weight loss of 25 lb (11.4 kg)
    b. A weight loss of 25 lb and galactorrhea
    c. Intense fear of obesity and a weight gain of 25 lb
    d. Disturbance in body image and an intense fear of gaining weight

65. A nursing diagnosis of disturbance in body image is indicative of which of the following disorders?
    a. Organic brain disorder
    b. Nutritional disorder
    c. Personality disorder
    d. Eating disorder

66. What is the key element in bulimia nervosa?
    a. Malnutrition
    b. Psychosis
    c. Binge-purge cycle
    d. Weight loss

67. Which of the following are signs and symptoms of bulimia nervosa?
    a. Binging-purging and skin changes
    b. Headaches and dehydration
    c. Dry, brittle hair; self-induced vomiting
    d. Stomachaches, binging-purging

68. A combination of therapies such as individual and group therapy, behavior modification, and nutritional counseling would be appropriate treatment for which of the following?
    a. Schizoaffective disorder
    b. Obsessive-compulsive disorder
    c. Anorexia nervosa
    d. Bipolar-affective disorder

CHAPTER 10

NURSING MANAGEMENT OF THE POTENTIALLY VIOLENT PATIENT

CHAPTER OBJECTIVE

After completing this chapter, the reader will be able to recognize a potentially violent situation and describe some nursing interventions that can be used to manage the situation.

LEARNING OBJECTIVES

After studying this chapter, the reader will be able to

1. Recognize three types of disorders that often are present in violent patients.

2. Choose the best way to manage a violent outburst.

3. Recognize the early warning signs of an escalating situation.

4. Define two types of restraints that can be used safely.

5. Indicate the nursing responsibilities related to use of chemical restraint procedures.

6. Recognize the procedure for safely restraining and managing an aggressive patient.

Rage, anger, and hostility are powerful and sometimes frightening emotions to have, as well as to confront in patients. The potential violence that may erupt because of these emotions can be quite scary for nursing personnel who work on general hospital units.

Although hospital-based violence occurs more often in psychiatric hospitals, it also occurs in nursing homes (high prevalence) and in general hospital units (low prevalence). In all cases, the targets of such violence tend to be nursing personnel. In one study (Jones, 1988) as many as 88% of violent occurrences in hospitals were directed toward members of the nursing staff.

Psychiatric nursing personnel are trained in the management of aggressive behavior and crisis situations involving escalation. Usually, nurses in a general hospital are not; often members of the security staff manage the occasional escalation of behavior. Members of the nursing staff should have some guidelines, however, for dealing with aggression, just as they do for a fire or other disaster. These guidelines should be based on a team approach with the security staff, because both security and nursing staff members are present and needed in these situations. Nursing home personnel, because of both the frequency of incidents and the delicate nature of some patients' conditions, certainly should have training in the management of potentially aggressive patients.

Patients considered more at risk for becoming aggressive are those who have had a violent outburst before. Aggressive patients most often have the following disorders:

- Organic brain syndromes/organic mental syndromes

- Substance abuse disorders

- Schizophrenia

- Borderline personality disorder

Incidents of violence are episodes or outbursts that involve hitting, choking, or generally assaulting another person; damaging property; throwing cups; smashing IV bottles; and so forth. Patients who resort to violence are extremely angry and frightened and feel out of control. Violent behavior is their attempt to respond to some stressful event, often one that they view as a direct personal threat. Patients who are psychotic or cognitively impaired because of a chemical or an organic process may misperceive normal hospital routines, which may include being handled physically by nursing personnel. Such patients may then strike out.

The best way to deal with a violent patient is to defuse the incident during the early stages of escalation. Watch for early warning signs and try to avoid a dangerous outburst. When this fails, your own safety and that of other patients and staff members, as well as that of the violent patient, must be considered.

The best method of action is to be prepared beforehand. Develop deescalation skills and learn hands-on skills for managing aggressive patients before aggression occurs. In-service education and training about the hospital's and the unit's plan for such an emergency cannot be undervalued.

EARLY WARNING SIGNS

Never overlook your own feelings of anxiety during a conversation or confrontation with a patient. If your intuition tells you that this patient may become dangerous or that the situation may be getting out of hand and potentially beyond your control, SEEK HELP EARLY. Consider yourself a good monitor of a potential crisis; pay attention to your gut reactions.

Anticipate potential problems. Know your patients' history as well as their current problems. Be alert to patients whose primary or secondary diagnoses are associated with a high degree of potential for violent occurrences. Patients who are potentially violent may exhibit the following behaviors:

- Become very loud; start shouting.

- Become physically tense; appear rigid and tight.

- Clench their teeth and hands.

- Be quite agitated, seemingly anxious and restless; perhaps pacing if mobile; seeming quite jittery.

- Have a labile mood, mostly anger.

Potentially violent patients often are demanding, argumentative, hostile, and perhaps challenging and blatantly threatening. This behavior may be directed toward staff members or toward the patients' family and friends, depending on the situation. A person seemingly in authority is often the recipient of this type of verbal abuse, although anyone who is in the way may be the target of a patient who cannot control himself or herself.

PRELIMINARY ACTIONS

Patients who are testy and seem to have the potential for violence should be managed carefully by the nursing staff. Nurses should avoid power struggles with these patients, to avoid confrontation. This conduct will help avoid escalating the patients' behavior and the situation. Give these patients choices and options. Do not be demanding and argumentative; perhaps some rules or procedures can be waived temporarily. Patients who are angry and potentially violent generally feel helpless and powerless. They need help with their self-control.

Alert other members of the nursing staff of a potential problem. Do not call on new and inexperienced staff members. Additional personnel should be available to help with a crisis. Never allow yourself to be alone and vulnerable with a potentially violent patient or trapped in a room away from the exit. Team up with another member of the staff when you see such a patient; there can be safety in numbers.

Open and consistent communication should be ongoing between staff members and between the patient and the staff. Talk to the patient. Try to find out what is precipitating this crisis. Ask what the patient would like done. How can the staff help? How can you, the nurse, help?

Before the situation gets out of control, check the environment. Look for potentially dangerous objects and remove them if possible. Items such as glasses, scissors, food utensils, and other breakable or sharp objects can be used as weapons.

Decrease the stimuli for the patient. The loud and unfamiliar noises of the hospital may be particularly stressful, or bright lights may be bothersome. Be careful when physical contact is needed in the course of nursing duties. Physical touch can be a trigger. Patients may misinterpret the contact and feel threatened with bodily harm, which they may need to defend themselves against. Delay procedures that may escalate a patient's potentially violent behavior.

WHEN VIOLENCE ERUPTS

If the potential for violence escalates, and a patient is behaving in a threatening manner, the nursing staff must take action quickly. Always seek aid in an emergency. Get help from the security staff, other nursing personnel, or any other hospital personnel who are available. Never attempt to manage a violent situation alone.

A patient who has a weapon should be disarmed by persons who are trained to do so. If the patient cannot be disarmed easily, your safety and that of others in the area must be considered.

Although you may be able to protect yourself with shields and barriers against knives, this may not be the case if a patient has a loaded gun.

The patient may need to be controlled externally with physical restraints or possibly medically restrained with tranquilizers. Some situations may call for both. When a patient needs to be subdued, it is preferable to use a team approach in handling the patient safely.

Chemical Restraint

Use of tranquilizing medications is one way of managing a patient's violent episode. The medications most often used are either the low-dose, high-potency antipsychotics such as haloperidol (Haldol) or the short-acting benzodiazepine lorazepam (Ativan). In some situations, patients may become violent as a result of psychosis and thereby need an antipsychotic. However, because danger to themselves or others is imminent, all will benefit by decreasing the patient's agitation as well. Such patients therefore are given both an antipsychotic and lorazepam.

Each general hospital has, or should have, some guidelines for the use of medications in this type of situation, and all nurses should be aware of this procedure. The medication orders may read as follows: Haldol 10 mg intramuscularly (IM) every hour until sedated and/or Ativan 2 mg IM for agitation. The antipsychotic medication is given as an initial dose, and the patient is observed at 15-min intervals. In some instances, medication may be given as often as every half hour until the violent episode is in check.

The patient may be quite willing to take the medication orally. The action of these drugs is slower, however, when they are taken orally. If the situation is moderate, the patient can be offered this alternative route.

The nursing responsibilities involved in handling a violent episode by medicating a patient with a potent pharmacologic agent include the following:

- Checking for or obtaining a physician's order

- Preparing the medication: capsules, tablets, or liquid; IM injection; or IV drip or butterfly infusion

- Assessing the patient's vital signs (e.g., blood pressure, pulse, and respiration) before giving the drugs

- Informing the patient of the procedure to follow and providing reassurance and support if needed

- After the medication has been administered, observing the patient and assessing for a decrease in signs and symptoms and for any untoward side effects

- Periodically checking the patient's vital signs

- Documenting the incident and the medications given by recording the information in the patient's chart or as the institution directs

Mechanical Restraint

Sometimes because of their physical or general medical condition, patients cannot take neuroleptic medications. Although episodes of violence to others may be rare in a general hospital, self-directed violence by psychotic or delirious patients does occur. Some situations may require that patients be restrained mechanically to prevent them from harming themselves or from leaving the hospital precipitously when leaving may be a significant threat to their health. Sometimes patients need both chemical and mechanical restraints.

As with protocols for using chemical restraint, each general hospital should have a procedure to follow for physically restraining a patient. One institution's rule of thumb for subduing an assaultive patient is to have one staff member available to hold each extremity and an additional staff member available to apply the restraints. The general recommendation is that five to six trained staff members are necessary for the hands-on management of a violent patient.

The patient is held by his or her arms and legs and walked, carried, or placed in as comfortable a position as possible, usually in a hospital bed with side rails up, and placed in wrist and ankle restraints. These restraints may be cotton, gauze, cloth, or leather, depending on the patient's size and strength.

In psychiatric facilities, patients who are restrained mechanically usually are placed in seclusion. Special rooms are set aside for just such an emergency. These rooms generally have no furniture except, perhaps, a mattress or bed and often are soundproof. They can be locked from the outside. A small window in the door allows staff members to check on the patient's safety and well-being. These rooms are stripped of all possible objects that could be used to cause harm to the patient (self-harm) or to others. They provide a quiet place for patients to regain some self-control; all stimuli are decreased.

General hospitals usually do not have such rooms available. Large hospitals with busy emergency departments may have a holding room designated for psychiatry that can be used for this type of seclusion.

When a patient is restrained mechanically in a general hospital, the number of staff members needed and the type of restraint required depend on the patient's size and strength and potential for violence. Ideally, one person should be in charge of a group of five or six staff members. If no one person is in charge, the possibility of mixing up messages, with everyone going in different directions, or having different ideas of what needs to be done and how to do it, can produce a disjointed effort, and the patient may escape and be harmed or do harm. The confusion that ensues when no one is in charge invariably adds to the patient's sense of being out of control and thus escalates the situation.

The best approach toward the patient is a uniform one. All staff members should move or walk toward the patient together. Sometimes this simple show of force, the sheer numbers, subdues a patient. To avoid confusion, before the approach is begun, the team leader should assign which staff member will hold which extremity. For maximal control, hold patients firmly just above or below their joints (elbows and knees) when walking them. Use the most secure hold you can. If you need to loosen a patient's grip on you, first try to tug the patient's thumb away gently; the rest of the hand will follow. The staff member or members who may be near the patient's head must be aware that the patient may try to bite them. Be alert.

Staff members should try to be calm themselves. Do not speak loudly; instead be firm and speak slowly, clearly, and precisely. A soft voice may have a quieting effect on the patient.

Whenever mechanical restraint is necessary, be firm. Do not negotiate with the patient, and do not confuse the patient with too many options. Remember, this patient is out of control. You may want to say something similar to the following: "We feel you are not in good control of yourself right now. We will help you calm down. You need to remain in this bed, and then we can talk."

Remember to check the room for potentially dangerous objects. Remove any watches, glasses, jewelry, shoes, and so forth that could be a hazard. Keep in mind that no place is absolutely free of danger. Patients have broken light bulbs and cut themselves with the shards. One patient used the cord in his pajama waist to hang himself. Be cautious and aware. Look around the area from the patient's eye level so you can see what the patient sees.

If the optimal number of staff members needed to subdue someone safely is not available, or if you are alone in a precarious situation, you may need to use a device as a blockade. You can use a blanket, a sheet, or even a mattress to take someone down to the floor initially or to protect yourself. This maneuver can buy you time or stun the patient temporarily until others arrive to help you apply restraints as needed. REMEMBER: For any of these techniques, training is essential to keep both you and the patient safe.

The safety of the patient and your own safety should be considered at all times. Try to present yourself as not being punitive but as attempting to help the patient regain some self-control over violent behavior.

Patients should be shown respect and allowed to maintain their dignity. Make sure everyone knows the patient's name and uses it. Avoid nicknames or expressions such as the following:

- Shut up, Mac!

- Calm down now, fella.

- Take it easy, grandpop.

Never underestimate the potential for violence. The only time I was ever assaulted was by a young woman who was my own age. She hit me over the head with her deodorant can. I was never threatened by a big man. Do not let preconceived notions and fantasies make you err about what type of person would or would not be a danger.

NURSING DIAGNOSES

The nursing diagnoses that are often considered with patients who are potentially violent are as follows:

- Risk for violence, self-directed or directed at others

- Ineffectual individual coping

- Fear

- Self-esteem disturbance

- Impaired social interactions

- Powerlessness

- Defensive coping

- Altered thought processes

NURSING INTERVENTIONS

The role of the nurse in the management of a potentially or actually violent patient will be found within the protocol, policy, or procedure manual of each institution. Within this framework, the following nursing interventions may apply:

- Anticipate a potential problem. Trust your judgment. Alert others of the potential problem.

- Assess the patient. Use good interpersonal skills, establish a rapport, and assess for the potentially violent occurrence.

- Assess the patient's coping skills and ability. Crisis intervention techniques may work early to prevent violent eruption.

- Use stress reduction techniques (e.g., deep breathing).

- Communicate verbally with the patient in a soft but firm voice. Attempt to foster a therapeutic relationship.

- Continually observe patients who are potentially dangerous to themselves or others.

- Monitor the situation for the safety of others and of yourself.

- Initiate or collaborate on a plan that includes a team approach to restraining a patient.

- Follow the individual institution's protocol, policy, or procedure for restraining a patient either mechanically or chemically.

- Document the violent incident and report it to all pertinent members of the health care team.

- After the patient has been restrained, plan future interventions by having a follow-up team meeting to discuss the effectiveness of the restraint procedure. Was it smooth, safe, and effective, or were there many glitches, patients not responding positively, or staff members hurt?

- Revise and review the protocol.

- In some states the law requires a legal hold if the patient is restrained with more than a Posey belt or soft restraints. In addition, restraints may necessitate one-to-one observation by staff. It is important to know your hospital's policy and what your state law requires.

CASE STUDY

A 58-year-old man, Mr. Anno, was admitted to a urologic unit for a transurethral resection for his benign prostatic hypertrophy. During the admission intake, Mr. Anno's daughter mentioned his mood swings. Mr. Anno spoke in broken English; Spanish was his native language.

The evening before his surgery, Mr. Anno spoke in an animated manner, in Spanish, to another patient. Twice the evening nurse came to Mr. Anno's bedside to calm him down and see what was wrong, because he was gesturing and muttering to himself, quite loudly at times. The physician on call was notified, and when he saw Mr. Anno, the patient was still animated but not as wild. The physician ordered a sedative, and said he would check again in an hour. Mr. Anno fell asleep in a short while. The rest of the evening shift was unremarkable.

Mr. Anno awoke about 6 a.m. and was given his preoperative medications. He was taken for surgery at 7 a.m. The surgery went well, with no complications. Mr. Anno had an unremarkable recovery, medically, and was returned to his unit at 2 p.m., where he was received by Ms. Kristen, his primary nurse.

Although he appeared somewhat sleepy, Mr. Anno was mumbling to himself and gesturing with his hands. Ms. Kristen became somewhat concerned when these behaviors seemed to increase and Mr. Anno's voice became louder. He then began to appear very tense, grimacing and clenching his fists. When Ms. Kristen approached him, he seemed angry with her, and she was confused as to why. Ms.Kristen reported her concerns to her head nurse: "I'm not sure what's going on with Mr. Anno, but I feel somewhat frightened of him." Ms. John, the head nurse, paged Mr. Anno's physician and attempted to get a Spanish language interpreter to come quickly to the unit.

In the meanwhile, Mr. Anno's postoperative wound needed checking, so both Ms. Kristen and Ms. John approached the patient's bedside. Much to their surprise, Mr. Anno began shouting loudly and attempted to pull out his IV line and catheter, seemingly to jump out of the bed. He picked up a wound dressing kit that was on his overbed tray and threw it at Ms. John. It hit her in the face, stunning her but not hurting her.

The two nurses then intervened appropriately in the following manner:

1. Ms. John announced that she would take charge.

2. A call for help from the rest of the unit's staff was made, and one of them was told to notify the security staff.

3. The other patients were removed from the area.

4. Ms. Kristen, Ms. John, and two nursing aides (one man and one woman) held Mr. Anno by his hands and feet.

5. Another nurse brought some mechanical soft restraints, and under Ms. John's direction, these were placed on the patient.

6. Mr. Anno's physician arrived, and after reviewing the situation, quickly ordered the following: Haloperidol 5 mg IM STAT to be followed by Haloperidol 5 mg IM every hour, until sedated.

7. The patient was told in Spanish about the medication and why he would receive some.

8. A staff member remained at the patient's bedside.

After this incident was under control, Ms. Kristen, Ms. John, Mr. Anno's physician, and the two nursing aides spent 20 min in a conference room reviewing the episode. A plan was made to confer with the family about Mr. Anno's mood swings, request a psychiatric evaluation, use Spanish-speaking personnel when available, and maintain close observation of this patient.

Although incidents of violence are not common in a general hospital, they can and do occur. It is important that all nurses have some education or training in the safe and appropriate use of precautions to follow for these untoward and least expected episodes.

EXAM QUESTIONS

CHAPTER 10
Questions 69–72

69. Defusing an incident is the best way to manage which of the following types of patients?

    a. A violent patient

    b. A patient who has an organic brain syndrome

    c. A hysterical patient

    d. A catatonic patient

70. Three types of disorders associated with violent patients are organic mental syndrome, substance abuse, and:

    a. Obsessive-compulsive disorder

    b. Bipolar affective illness

    c. Schizophrenia

    d. Paranoia

71. Which of the following may be an early warning sign of a violent episode?

    a. Increases in blood pressure, pulse rate, and respirations

    b. Hysterical laughing and agitation

    c. Elevated lithium levels

    d. Yelling, teeth clenching, and angry appearance

72. What is the recommended number of staff members needed to restrain a patient safely?

    a. One to two

    b. Two to four

    c. Five to six

    d. Eight to nine

CHAPTER 11

NURSING MANAGEMENT OF THE NONCOMPLIANT PATIENT

CHAPTER OBJECTIVE

After completing this chapter, the reader will be able to recognize the major risk factors for noncompliance by patients and specify interventions to increase compliance.

LEARNING OBJECTIVES

After studying this chapter, the reader will be able to

1. Describe the Health Belief Model of noncompliance.

2. Specify risk factors for noncompliance.

3. Recognize characteristics of the elderly that influence compliance.

4. Correctly specify diagnoses related to noncompliance.

5. Indicate the phases of the cycle of noncompliance that occurs between nurse and patient.

6. Recognize the best tools nurses can use in dealing with noncompliance in patients.

7. Recognize risk factors for departures from the hospital that are against medical advice.

8. Give a good example of a possible conflict between the principle of personal freedom and the principle of social responsibility.

9. Recognize the defining characteristics of a competent patient.

INTRODUCTION

A diabetic patient has been instructed about dietary restrictions and still eats foods that are not allowed. A patient with emphysema finds every opportunity to smoke. A pregnant mother with signs of premature labor gets up from recommended bed rest to fix her family's dinner.

Patients are often noncompliant with their treatment regimens. The noncompliant patient presents a unique challenge in patient care. Dealing with noncompliance may present some of the most difficult and, at the same time, rewarding experiences for nurses.

The concept of noncompliance is a subject of debate in health care. At issue is the right of the patient to choose a treatment course that is different from the recommendations of the health care team. Nurses are in a pivotal role to affect the course of treatment.

Noncompliance is an emotionally laden issue for many health care providers. Changes in health care have created an environment in which the roles of providers, the demands and needs of consumers, and legal standards are continually evolving. Nurses must have a strong nursing philosophy and solid nursing skills to guide them through the dilemmas that have become a frequent occurrence in the general hospital setting. Noncompliance is often a factor in those dilemmas.

DEFINITIONS

What is noncompliance? The NANDA (1994) definition of noncompliance is "a person's informed decision not to adhere to a therapeutic recommendation."

Many think, however. that compliance implies a power differential in the relationship between a patient and the health care provider. Edel (1985), for example, describes the compliance relationship as one in which "one individual behaves in accordance with directives supported by another individual's power. Those who have power, control and manipulate means in such a way that others find that following their directives is rewarding, while not doing so brings about deprivation."

Although this definition may be distasteful to many nurses, it may more accurately reflect the reality for patients. Rewards that a nurse might give to a compliant patient might include a smile, more time spent in the patient's room, or a quicker response to the patient's call light. Nurses are usually unwilling to think that they may be depriving the patient of anything. However, they can help noncompliant patients move toward compliance by planning a course of behavior.

IMPACT AND PREVALENCE

Estimates of the extent of noncompliance vary widely, but most research indicates that an average of one third of all patients are noncompliant with their treatment regimen (e.g., Kaplan & Sadock, 1991). Being able to predict which patients will comply with recommendations and which ones will not would be useful. Early intervention could then help patients who are at risk for noncompliance.

Because information on noncompliance is needed to make decisions about allocation of health care resources, studies on this issue focus on methods to pinpoint who will be compliant. In the current climate of limited health care dollars, many health care professionals are anticipating (and in some specialties are already dealing with) the prospect of having to choose who receives limited health care resources. However, currently we cannot accurately predict which patients will be compliant.

Cummings et al. (1982) compared ratings by nurses, objective laboratory indicators, and self-report methods in a study of compliance in dialysis patients. The most valid approach was ratings by nurses, although only 50% of the time. These findings highlight the integral role of the nurse-patient relationship in recognizing problems with compliance. Other predictors of compliance have variable validity. Patients tend to overstate their compliance. Physicians are able to predict compliance at only chance levels of accuracy (Cummings et al., 1984).

Compliance is usually associated with optimal health, although no research findings support this point of view. In the past 25 years, however, a shift has occurred from medically directed treatment regimens to an emphasis on the patient as an active consumer and decision maker. The nurse's role as advocate and facilitator for patients and families negotiating health care systems is a pivotal one. The difference between compliance and noncompliance may be due to the skilled observations and interventions of the nurse.

THE PURPOSE AND MEANING OF NONCOMPLIANCE

All behavior has meaning. In hospitals, patients are separated from their homes and families. They are in a strange environment and are assuming a new role. They are in crisis, and therefore their interactions with the environment and the people in it are stressed. Their coping mechanisms may be impaired.

Nurses are familiar with the hospital environment and may forget that patients can be unsure and anxious. Patients are asked to take off their clothes and to confine their movement to restricted areas. They are allowed to feed themselves when hospital routine says it is time to eat and not when they are hungry. The list of challenges that a patient encounters in the hospital can be endless.

Most patients are also quite fearful of pain, and in the hospital, a nurse is often in control of measures to alleviate pain. In fact, most patients perceive that nurses are in control of many factors that directly affect the patients' welfare. If asked, many patients state that they are afraid that if they do not behave in a certain way, the nurse will "retaliate."

If we imagine what our own reactions might be if we were forced to enter such an environment, the compliance-noncompliance issue has new meaning. In order to promote compliance, hospitalization must become an experience in which patients maintain control over most of what happens to them. Providers are finding new ways to alleviate the dilemmas that patients face when hospitalized. An example is the PCA pump for self-administration of pain medication. Use of this device reduces the patient's dependence on the nurse for comfort and, in many cases, reduces anxiety about pain control.

Many attempts have been made to create a conceptual model of compliance that will enable health care providers to predict and understand patients' behavior. The Health Belief Model offers some understanding of the phenomenon of compliance. The model proposes reasons for people's varied and unique responses to illness. The significance of this model is that a patient's choices depend on his or her beliefs and not necessarily on the medical evaluation of the situation.

The model postulates that people choose health actions when they are faced with a threat to their health. The actions they choose depend on three perceptions (Cummings et al., 1984):

1. The severity of the health threat

2. How directly they feel the health action will reduce the health threat

3. What the cost will be in their life if they take the health action

Compliance, therefore, is a function of both the patient's belief system and his or her understanding of the disease and its treatment. For many patients, noncompliance may be their perception that the illness is less of a problem than the treatment is.

Thorne (1990) analyzed data from interviews with 77 patients and family members dealing with chronic illness. She concluded that the word *noncompliance* was an accurate description of the power structures of health care systems and the systems' inability to accommodate the unique needs of each family. Her participants made purposeful decisions to be noncompliant with the recommendations of those systems.

Thorne found three distinct categories of noncompliance:

1. Simple modification of treatment regimens

2. Selective noncompliance, in which certain recommendations were rejected and others were followed

3. Agreeing, with no intention of following through

Her respondents cited an increasing sense of independence and responsibility associated with their noncompliance. In addition, most of them had experienced a situation or a series of events that led to a loss of confidence in the "experts." Her findings suggest that in some cases, noncompliance may be a reasonable and healthy assertion of independence.

The respondents realized that "health care professionals operate from a fixed set of beliefs rather than from a foundation of universal truths" and noticed that such beliefs were subject to considerable human interpretation. No health care provider is perfect and infallible. In some situations, it may be appropriate for patients to choose purposeful noncompliance.

Still another view of noncompliance is that the health care provider who applies the label may be blind to the real issues. Often, skilled assessment is required to uncover the reasons for a patient's non-compliance. If the health care provider does not take the time or does not have the skills to truly understand the patient's view of the illness and treatment recommendations, the patient is more likely to be noncompliant.

Noncompliance, then, is a complex problem. The label probably covers a variety of issues. The nursing diagnosis of noncompliance should be used only after careful exploration of the patient's particular situation and his or her attitudes and beliefs.

RISK FACTORS

Patients' characteristics and environment influence the likelihood that they will be compliant or noncompliant. Knowledge of risk factors can help nurses be more aware of the possibility that a patient may have difficulties being compliant. Risk factors are most helpful when used to prevent possible problems.

Social Risk Factors

The social spheres that most affect a patient's health behaviors are as follows:

1. Family, significant others
2. Relationships with health care providers
3. Cultural or ethnic group
4. Religious community or beliefs

Family behaviors can influence noncompli-ance. Hemodialysis patients who reported fewer family problems were more compliant with their treatment regimens than patients who reported more problems. In another study (Cummings et al., 1982), patients who received more assistance from their spouses (in general and in health matters) had higher compliance than patients who received less assistance.

Compliance has been positively correlated with the quality of communication among family mem-bers of hemodialysis patients. Effective human communication systems appear to protect patients from noncompliance. Social isolation also con-tributes to noncompliance (Cummings et al., 1982).

However, social support is not always a moti-vating factor (Padrick, 1986). It is important to remember that the family's role, as well as the nurse's, is to support the patient's compliance, not to enforce it (King, 1990). Ultimately, the decision to be compliant is the patient's.

Research has shown that patients tend to con-form to the expectations of their health care provider (Cummings et al., 1982). However, this tendency may occur only at certain times. The rela-tionship between care provider and patient may have a developmental sequence. Perhaps at a cer-tain point in the relationship, the patient is more prone to be noncompliant.

Some evidence also indicates that compliance in patients with chronic illnesses has predictable phases. Patients tend to be very compliant in the beginning of the illness and become less compliant over time.

The mutuality of expectations of patients and health care providers is important. One study (Young, 1986) found that patients had expectations of providers. If these expectations were not met, the patients had a lower level of compliance. In addition, these impressions were formed in the first moments of the patient's exposure to the health care system. Nurses and hospitals would be wise to focus on the admission process to make it a posi-tive experience, because it will shape the ongoing relationship with the patient.

The patient's perceptions about the care provider are important also. If the patient perceives the provider as interested, concerned, and caring, then compliance is higher (McCord, 1986). This finding emphasizes the importance of the interpersonal connection between the patient and the nurse.

A patient's cultural or religious beliefs and practices may prohibit compliance with a treatment regimen. Some religions view the use of certain types of medical interventions as a lack of faith in God, and those procedures are therefore prohibited. Some cultures have lay healers, and the patient may wish to combine the healer's cures with medical treatment. Many cultures view healing as a family affair, and therefore the family will need to be always present and involved in the patient's care. Nurses must try to understand and appreciate the importance of these practices in order to help patients be compliant.

Socioeconomic status and educational level are not related to compliance. In addition, race and sex do not affect compliance levels (McCord, 1986). The very young and the elderly are more likely than other age groups to be noncompliant.

Environmental Risk Factors

The care setting can influence compliance. The most common factors are comfort issues and ease of access, including transportation. The needs of physically impaired patients must be considered carefully.

For example, an elderly person who has been directed to return to the clinic after a surgical admission may not keep this appointment. The patient may not have transportation, the parking may be too remote for him or her to walk from the car to the building, or the stairs may be too much for him or her to handle. If there is little to motivate the patient's return, these environmental obstacles will result in noncompliance.

A significant concern is limited income. Patients may have hospitalization coverage but few funds to follow through on recommendations after discharge. A patient who must choose between feeding his or her family and buying blood pressure medicine has no choice at all. Examining patients' finances with them and planning realistic health care choices together can be helpful.

Psychological Risk Factors

The most important psychological risk factors include the following:

- Cognitive abilities
- Mental status
- Denial and anxiety
- Addictions
- Depression
- Past experiences

Psychological and cognitive factors may influence compliance. To be able to comply, patients must understand the information presented to them. In addition, the patient's judgment may influence the choice to comply.

Patients with cognitive deficits may not be able to learn. Patients must be capable of concentrating and of practicing new behaviors and have an adequate attention span to tolerate the learning process. In any event, recommendations must be aimed at the patient's learning level to be effective.

Similarly, patients with changes in mental status will be unable to integrate new learning material effectively. In addition, their judgment may be significantly impaired. A thorough mental status examination is needed if there is any indication that a patient's mental status is compromised.

On the first day after surgery, a patient may appear to be oriented enough for patient teaching but later often will remember only that the nurse had visited. Little of the information given to the patient will be retained. Patients often express frustration about this problem.

Patients who are in denial have little reason to

retain treatment information. They do not believe that their illness is significant, so treatment recommendations are seen as unnecessary. Denial is a defense against uncomfortable feelings. Patients may be too frightened by their illness to be able to accept it.

Denial is a normal part of grieving and sometimes occurs in people when they find out they have a terminal illness. Illness and hospitalization involve losses for people regardless of the prognosis, and denial may be part of any patient's presentation. People in denial need time to adjust and an opportunity to discuss their difficult feelings.

Some patients use denial as a primary and consistent defense, however, and become much more anxious when provided with information. They often have a family member assume the role of decision maker in the course of their illness. The level of compliance in such patients is variable.

Anxiety reduces anyone's ability to process information or to make decisions. An anxious patient might behave in a number of ways, including anger, complaining, demanding, withdrawing, or even crying. Reducing the anxiety will aid in compliance. Many patients are fearful of the unknown. Education often allays these fears.

Addictions affect compliance because they take top priority in the addicted person's life. If the treatment regimen interferes in any way with the addictive behavior, the patient will not be compliant until the addiction is treated. The classic example of this is the alcoholic who has cirrhosis. The recommended treatment is abstinence from alcohol, but few alcoholics can accomplish this without professional intervention.

Depression is significantly related to lowered compliance (King, 1990). A person who is clinically depressed will not take in information or make decisions as well as one who is not depressed. Depressed persons have low self-esteem and feelings of hopelessness that can interfere with

their ability to follow a regimen to better their health.

Depression is the most common mental health problem in the United States. Unfortunately, although it is probably the easiest to treat, it is the least treated, and depressed patients are often overlooked. Nurses are in an ideal position to observe depressed behavior and initiate further evaluation. Depressed patients need careful observation, adequate sleep, as much exercise as possible, and expert intervention. Psychiatrists, clinical psychologists, clinical social workers, and psychiatric clinical nurse specialists are some of the trained practitioners who can be called on to intervene with depressed patients.

Finally, each patient enters the health care system with ideas and beliefs that affect the course of the current hospitalization. Previous experiences that were negative can affect a patient's expectations. If a patient enters the system expecting the worst, chances are good that health care recommendations will not be viewed in a positive light.

Determining risk factors early in treatment enables nurses to intervene effectively. Nurses are in the best position to use their skills to develop a care plan with the patient that maximizes compliance. In the same way, knowledge of risk factors can enhance discharge planning.

RELATED CONCEPTS

Two concepts closely related to the issue of noncompliance are age and knowledge. Health care providers rely heavily on education to increase compliance, and therefore an examination of the relationship between the two is useful. In addition, elderly patients have many physiologic and situational factors that affect compliance. It is worth examining their special needs to understand their risk for noncompliance.

Knowledge

Patient education receives a great deal of emphasis in nursing. Because teaching is important, several issues should be considered when nurses explore educational deficits in patients. Some of the assumptions about teaching may not be valid.

One study found that compliance rates had no relationship to increased knowledge. Other studies found that specific educational programs had an impact on patients' adherence to treatment regimens. Young (1986) concluded that "education is a viable strategy but should not be used as the only intervention for increasing compliance."

Young has also described some characteristics of learners. Within 5 min people forget approximately half of the statements made to them by health care professionals. They remember only the first third of the information. Written information fosters compliance, but it must be written at the fourth-grade level. As the complexity of information increases, compliance decreases. Some people are visual learners and benefit from use of drawings, charts, practice sessions, and so on.

These findings remind us that teaching should be brief and focused. Complex information should be broken into smaller, understandable parts whenever possible. It is helpful to simplify teaching material as much as possible.

In addition, some patients apparently just do not want to know. These patients find information anxiety producing instead of comforting. They are challenges, because they require a different approach that does not rely heavily on patient teaching. The nurse must be more direct and rely on family members to assist in compliance.

Age

The estimated rate of noncompliance for the elderly is 50%. They are more at risk for noncompliance than other adult patients are. In general, the elderly are less informed than other age groups about drugs and diseases (Welch-McCaffrey, 1986).

Because of their unique needs, older patients present a challenge in compliance. Their hearing, vision, and cognitive functioning are likely to be impaired in some way. These handicaps make changes in behavior difficult.

Most patients 60 years and older require correction of vision. In the over 70 age bracket, almost 15% are considered legally blind. Of those 80 and over, 36% have cataracts. In addition, the lens of the eye yellows with age, making it difficult to distinguish colors (King, 1990). These impairments make self-administration of medications particularly difficult.

Almost one third of all people 65–79 years old have significant hearing impairment. In addition, the ability to think abstractly slows with age, and information is not absorbed as quickly (King, 1990). In the elderly, recall is best when material is given verbally. Information must be delivered slowly and audibly.

Depression is common in the elderly. It often goes undetected and untreated. Depression lessens the ability of older patients to adapt to changes in their life-style.

The elderly also must deal with a decrease in manual dexterity (King, 1990). Seemingly simple tasks such as picking up a pill become difficult. Plans for self-treatment must take this loss in dexterity into account.

Older people often find that their social support systems are shrinking. Friends and relatives may be ill, dying, or making changes in living arrangements. The resulting isolation can affect compliance.

The number of medications prescribed for older patients can be a problem. At least one fourth of the elderly recently discharged from hospitals have six or more prescriptions that require self-administration. Health care providers know that the more prescription medications a person must contend with, the lower is the person's compliance. If more than three drugs are prescribed for any patient, the risk for noncompliance increases (Kaplan & Sadock, 1991).

It is easy to see why the noncompliance rates for the elderly are high. This population is also less likely to be assertive about their needs with health care providers. The elderly constitute a major part of general care patients today. Nurses need to be sensitive to the unique needs of this age group.

IS NONCOMPLIANCE AN APPROPRIATE DIAGNOSIS?

Although it has been the subject of much debate, noncompliance remains a NANDA-approved nursing diagnosis. Research has shown that the meaning of this NANDA diagnosis is one of the most unclear. Although 52% of respondents in one study reported using the diagnosis, they could not find a consensus definition (Whitley, 1991). It may be that noncompliance is many things and not a specific syndrome. NANDA (1994) characterizes noncompliance as "behavior indicative of failure to adhere (by direct observation or by statements of patient or significant others); objective tests (physiological measures, detection of markers); evidence of development of complications; evidence of exacerbation of symptoms; failure to keep appointments; failure to progress."

Nurses have argued that the diagnosis of noncompliance labels the patient negatively. It is true that the behavior of care providers seems to be different with patients labeled as noncompliant. In practice, nurses often withdraw from these patients.

Finally, focusing on noncompliance places the emphasis on the patient's behavior instead of on a mutual process with the nurse. The label implies aberrant behavior on the part of the patient. Some argue that the person who needs to change his or her behavior is the care provider.

When the nursing diagnosis is noncompliance, the specific therapeutic recommendation that the patient is not complying with should be specified. Related diagnoses include the following:

- Self-care deficit
- Anxiety
- Powerlessness
- Knowledge deficit
- Compromised family coping
- Ineffective individual coping

STRATEGIES AND INTERVENTIONS

The Nurse's Reaction to the Noncompliant Patient

The nurse's willingness to look at his or her attitudes and feelings is of primary importance in dealing with noncompliant patients. The identity of nursing is closely tied to the concepts of helping, caring, and service. When a patient appears to reject a nurse's expertise in promoting wellness, the nurse must deal with many intense and conflicting emotions.

Many nurses state that they would prefer to spend their time with patients who want to get well and are motivated to do so rather than with a patient who does not comply with his or her treatment plan. They express anger that the patient is "wasting" a bed, precious resources, or nurses' time.

Sometimes, this anger leads to withdrawal of services to that patient. A nurse may avoid going in the patient's room or omit teaching the patient, because "the patient isn't going to do it anyway."

Ironically, the person who most needs assistance is left without support (Padrick, 1986).

At times, nurses may feel unable to "allow" a patient to be noncompliant. This situation might occur when the nurse has some commonalty with the patient, such as being the same age as the patient or having a parent who died of the disease the patient has. Nurses who feel powerless in the face of a patient's noncompliance may push the patient to comply while assuming decision-making responsibilities that belong to the patient.

Behavior is driven by feelings that arise in response to the patient's noncompliant behavior. It is important to note, however, that the patient's needs are not adequately met. The patient is overlooked, because the nurse's actions are based on the nurse's feelings and not on the patient's needs.

Furthermore, a patient may be quite satisfied with the nurse's behavior. Depending on the reasons for the noncompliance, the patient may be quite happy to be left alone or to be overly dependent on the nurse. More likely, however, the patient recognizes that his or her real health care needs go undetected.

This behavior becomes a cycle:

1. Patient is noncompliant.
2. Nurse feels angry, powerless, and so forth.
3. Nurse withdraws or becomes overactive.
4. Patient's needs go unmet.

Nurses can stop the cycle by doing the following:

- Becoming aware of their feelings.
- Doing a nursing assessment.
- Using care planning as a mutual process.

Awareness of feelings is an individual as well as a group process. Nurses who can recognize, for instance, that noncompliance makes them angry can begin to understand their behaviors and make changes. It is also helpful to talk with other nurses about similar feelings. It must be acceptable for nurses to share their frustrations, so that the frustrations are not acted out in interactions with patients.

Equally important is an orientation to patient care that values mutual development of agreed on goals. Care planning is a negotiation between the nurse, who has expert knowledge about what could be done, and the patient, who has expert knowledge about what will be done. A truly skilled nurse will search for the compromise that will work for the patient and will maximize the patient's health. Compliance can be improved by "asking patients directly to describe what they themselves believe is wrong with them [and] what they believe should be done" (Kaplan & Sadock, 1991).

Finally, a thorough assessment can uncover all sorts of removable obstacles to a patient's compliance. This step does require some extra time in establishing a relationship with the patient in which he or she will feel comfortable in explaining his or her unique situation. Noncompliant patients may be "burned-out" patients who require different strategies (Padrick, 1986) and a stretch from the nurse's usual practice.

Strategies for Helping Patients Make Life-Style Changes

Health promotion has been defined as "activities directed toward sustaining or increasing the level of well-being, self-actualization and personal fulfillment of a given individual or group. Health promotion, for most persons involves life-style changes" (Clark, 1986). Life-style changes are, perhaps, the most difficult changes a person can attempt. They often include diet, exercise, the use of drugs (prescribed or illicit), activity level, cutting back on work time, and so on.

Patients can be assisted in making life-style changes. The amount of change required is related to the level of compliance (Cummings et al., 1982). Faced with enormous change, many people give up. They are more likely to succeed if changes are broken down into manageable pieces.

The definition of manageable is unique to each person and may have to be negotiated several times. People often say they will change their behavior but find themselves unable to follow through. It is helpful if the patient is encouraged to renegotiate the steps in an effort to change.

The area of most promise in uncovering obstacles to compliance is what Cummings et al. (1982) term *situational factors*. These are events in the patient's daily life that create an environment for noncompliance. For example, the patient lets a prescription run out and misses doses before he or she is able to get to the pharmacy. Or the patient on a limited diet is at a restaurant that cannot meet the requirements of the diet.

Situational factors are best dealt with through anticipatory planning. A conversation with the patient about the possibility of these events and how to prepare for them can help in compliance. A patient on a restricted diet, for example, is asked to consider eating at home until he or she is familiar with the diet. The patient is also given ideas about what to order in a restaurant that would be within the requirements. He or she may feel uncomfortable explaining the diet to friends. Role playing situations such as these are helpful.

It is helpful to remember that you must repeat things over and over again before the patient will retain them. A good plan is to decide on one or two major points that you want to discuss. State them clearly in the beginning of the meeting with the patient. Reinforce them by referring to them several times during the interaction. Finally, include them in a summary statement to the patient.

A Special Case: The Patient Who Signs Out Against Medical Advice

Leaving the hospital against medical advice may be an extreme example of noncompliance. Nurses and physicians alike react strongly to this statement on the part of the patient. Health care providers may attempt to cajole or coerce the patient into staying. In this case, there are often real concerns about the patient's safety and the providers' obligations to the patient.

Leaving the hospital against medical advice is rarely a spontaneous act. There are often warning signals or repeated conflictual interactions with staff members before the patient actually signs out. Patients at greater risk for leaving have the following characteristics (Hackett & Stern, 1987):

- A history of leaving the hospital against medical advice

- Alcoholism or drug addiction (22–42% of patients who leave under such circumstances are addicted)

- A significant disturbance in the relationship between the health care provider and the patient

Patients should be free to leave as long as their judgment is good and they are not endangering their life. Ninety-four percent of patients who leave against medical advice return to the hospital. It is not appropriate to medicate a nonpsychotic patient who is threatening to leave against medical advice. Using drugs as chemical restraints in this manner is questionable from a legal standpoint. In addition, doing so will sever the already tenuous relationship with the patient (Hackett & Stern, 1987).

CASE STUDY

Mr. Scovil is a 60-year-old man who was admitted to the hospital after he fell and broke his hip. He had been helpless at home for several hours after the fall, because his wife was at work. On the day of admission, surgical repair was performed with the insertion of a nail and plate.

After surgery, Mr. Scovil was disoriented for several days. He was confused and belligerent and had visual hallucinations, and physical restraint was required part of this time. His blood pressure and pulse rate were high.

When his mental status cleared, his physical progression through the postoperative period was smooth. The incision healed with no excessive redness or swelling. His vital signs became stable.

It was difficult to develop a pain management regimen that enabled Mr. Scovil to experience pain relief. He was unwilling to practice coughing or deep breathing as ordered. It was a constant struggle to get him to ambulate, although he had been taught the dangers of immobility many times.

His wife and children rarely visited and were unwilling to talk with staff members. Mr. Scovil reported that he had not worked for many years and relied on his wife financially. He gave vague reasons for this situation, stating that he had been laid off and that there were never any jobs in his field of construction.

The nursing staff began to be concerned as time passed and Mr. Scovil did not appear to be assuming responsibility for his recovery. He, on the other hand, was eager to return home and pressured his physician to let him go prematurely. The staff called a patient care conference to discuss the discharge plans for Mr. Scovil.

During the conference, several of the nurses on the evening shift expressed concern that Mr. Scovil would not be well taken care of if he were to return home at this time. They had met his wife because she visited in the evening after work. They described her as "cold" and "mean." They were sure that she would provide no assistance to Mr. Scovil, who would be forced to fend for himself at home.

The night nurses described ongoing episodes of insomnia that the patient had experienced since his admission. One of the nurses had found Mr. Scovil attempting to smoke in his room. She stated that he drank cup after cup of coffee whenever he could. They thought that he was simply a noncompliant patient and should be discharged as soon as possible with home care assistance.

One of the nurses mentioned the possibility that Mr. Scovil might be alcoholic. She cited the delirious episode after admission, his low pain tolerance, and the dysfunction in the family as possible indicators that he might have a substance abuse problem. The physician added that the hypertensive episode after surgery and the insomnia supported that assessment.

The social worker remembered that Mr. Scovil's wife had bitterly discussed with her his lack of employment and his numerous falls. The social worker admitted that she had focused on the wife's hostility instead of on the possibility of alcoholism. She added that the behavioral habits of smoking and excessive coffee drinking have been linked to alcoholism.

It was agreed that the social worker would meet again with the wife and discuss the possibility that Mr. Scovil was alcoholic. With the information from that interview, it was easier to approach Mr. Scovil about his problem. He was referred for treatment of a substance abuse problem.

The evening staff nurses who described the patient's wife as cold and mean were clearly angry. If they had examined their feelings closely, they might have discovered that they were actually angry at the patient for his unwillingness to participate in recovery. It is often easier to be angry at a healthy, and distant, family member. It may be difficult for nurses to accept that they are angry at a patient who is ill and whom they see on a daily basis.

The night nurses felt little compassion for this patient. They were most likely dealing with feelings of powerlessness. Mr. Scovil was a patient who ignored the rules and the health care advice offered to him. Powerlessness is difficult for anyone to feel and is most often masked by anger and rejection.

Most of the issues of noncompliance in this

case study were attributable to the untreated chemical dependency. Mr. Scovil was unable to be compliant because of this addiction. If he were discharged home without treatment of the problem, his chances of a successful recovery would have been low. In addition, his alcoholism would have placed him at risk for more falls and other physical problems.

LEGAL AND ETHICAL ISSUES

Health care professionals are faced with increasingly complex situations in which the patient's wishes may deviate from the treatment recommendations. Some ethical guidelines can help nurses choose a response to a patient who is noncompliant. In addition, to practice within the law, nurses must be aware of legal guidelines. This area of health care is changing quickly. Nurses need to be clear about their obligations to patients and be knowledgeable about patients' rights.

Rights of the Patient

Inviolability is the fundamental right of every individual to be left alone. The U.S. Constitution and Bill of Rights are based on this principle, which is one of the clearest principles in common law (Burckhardt, 1986). The individual should have authority over what happens to his or her body.

In practice, however, the situation is not always so clear. In some instances, individual rights may interfere with the rights of others. In addition, fluctuations in public sentiment may affect the decisions made by practitioners and institutions.

Ethicists differ on their orientation to the dilemmas that health care professionals face. The concept of personal freedom can become unclear when the perspective is one of social responsibility. Some ethicists believe that people have both individual autonomy and responsibilities to one another.

The issue of mandatory testing for communicable diseases illustrates the dilemma of conflicting principles. Inviolability would guarantee the individual the right to refuse such testing. The principle of social responsibility would support mandatory testing, because the individual has the obligation to participate to protect others.

Burckhardt (1986) has described the widespread paternalism apparent in the medical model. Some might add that nursing has its own form of paternalism. The patient is treated as if he or she were a dependent, and the health care professional assumes a parental role as the "authority."

The following characterization of paternalism might sound familiar to nurses: The physician (in this case) will behave in such a way that

- The patient's freedom of action or information is interfered with.

- The physician may violate a moral rule of truthfulness by allowing deliberate misinformation.

- These behaviors are justified because they are in "the best interest" of the patient.

Paternalism interferes with patients' rights.

Legal Concerns

One legal issue that affects the nurse's part in compliance is the issue of competence. A patient is competent if he or she is able to participate in making decisions. A competent patient enters freely, without coercion, into a relationship with a health care provider who offers services to the patient.

The patient must be capable of understanding information about the offered services. For example, patients must be able to hear and understand the nature of their illness and the treatment alternatives available. Equally important is an understanding of the consequences of any decision the patient might make about these alternatives.

Patients are presumed to be competent. This assumption means that the burden of proving incompetence belongs to parties other than the patient. Unless otherwise indicated, we assume patients are making competent choices about their health care.

At times, however, patients may be caught in a frustrating contradiction between the issues of compliance and competence. A patient may refuse a treatment recommendation. Health care professionals may label the patient incompetent because of the refusal. In other words, the patient has made an informed decision and is cognitively capable of making the decision. However, because the patient has made the "wrong" decision, he or she is viewed as incompetent.

The validity of rationality (or the degree of rationality of the decision) as a determinant of competence is questionable. It is a subject of debate in the field of psychiatry (Pomerantz & de Nesnera, 1991). Often, the patient's decision is viewed as rational only if it coincides with the care provider's opinion.

Special Cases

Rights of pregnant women. Pregnancy offers a unique slant to the issue of patients' rights. For some people, the fact that the fetus is affected by the mother's behavior alters the mother's right to personal freedom. The legal system has increasingly overridden the right of the pregnant mother to disregard medical advice.

The legal basis for these decisions is weak. However, societal support for protecting the unborn fetus can result in disregard for the rights of the pregnant woman. The current debate over the rights of the unborn fetus versus the rights of the mother evokes intense emotions.

Withholding nutrition. There is little consensus on the ethics of withholding or withdrawing nutrition from patients. When a patient chooses to refuse nutrition, it is often difficult for health care

providers to honor this wish.

Nurses may be concerned about participating in behavior that will lead to hunger or thirst in the patient. It is important to remember that providing artificial nutrition and hydration do not necessarily reduce these sensations. Ice chips, good oral care, and lubricating the patient's lips may provide more comfort than artificial hydration, for example (Wurzbach, 1991).

In some ethical configurations, a distinction is made between allowing a patient to die and killing a patient. The difference lies with the intent of one's actions. Nutrition may be withheld on the premise that it will prolong life and thus prolong suffering. This is different from starving a patient with the intent to kill him or her.

Others argue that the finality of the act of withholding nutrition makes the act untenable. Starvation always leads to death, and therefore, they argue, health care providers should never withhold nourishment from a patient (Wurzbach, 1991). This is a difficult dilemma in health care.

The American Nurses Association's position on this subject is that nurses should provide food and fluid except in these cases:

1. When patients would be more harmed by receiving than by withholding of food and fluid

2. When competent patients refuse for "good reasons"

3. When the provision of food and fluid would inflict suffering that is not outweighed by an important long-term benefit

Furthermore, the Association suggests that the nurse err on the side of continuing nutrition and hydration even when these measures do not clearly provide benefit to the patient (Wurzbach, 1991).

It is imperative that every nurse be familiar with the legalities about patients' right to refuse treatment. In addition, careful thought concerning the nurse's own ethical position on these issues is necessary. The answers are not always clear in the increasingly complex environment of health care today.

SUMMARY

Noncompliance is a common behavior of people who are ill. Patients who are noncompliant present a challenge to the nurse. Nurses have an important role in helping patients recognize and change noncompliant behavior.

Few people agree on the definition of noncompliance. It is agreed that the noncompliant patient is not following treatment directives. The disagreement focuses on whether a power differential in the provider-patient relationship contributes to the patient's behavior.

Health care providers often react intensely to a noncompliant patient. The feelings evoked by the patient's behavior may change the nurse's approach to the patient. The nurse may withdraw or become overactive in the patient's care.

Early intervention is helpful in ending noncompliance. Currently, we cannot predict accurately which patients will be noncompliant. Among the members of the health care team, however, nurses appear to be the most able to recognize noncompliance.

Noncompliance has meaning in the patient's life. The nurse must be able to carefully assess the patient's situation to understand this meaning. In this way, obstacles to compliance can be uncovered and dealt with.

The Health Belief Model provides a way to understand but not predict noncompliance. This model focuses on the patient's beliefs and not the medical reality of the illness. For compliance to occur, the treatment must be less of a problem than the illness is.

Noncompliance can take many forms. Patients may make small changes in the treatment prescribed. They may reject whole recommendations while following some. Finally, some patients agree to follow health care advice when they have no intention of doing so.

Patients have reported a disillusionment with health care providers. Unmet expectations may predispose a patient to noncompliant behavior. The relationship between the patient and the health care provider has an important affect on the patient's health behaviors.

Social, environmental, and psychological risk factors seem to be associated with noncompliant behavior. Knowledge of a patient's risk factors is helpful in preventing potential problems.

Nurses should be willing to examine their feelings about noncompliance. A patient who appears to be rejecting treatment recommendations can evoke many conflicting emotions. If the nurse is aware, the feelings do not have to interfere with effective interactions with the patient. Remembering that compliance "depends on the specific clinical situation, the nature of the illness, and the treatment program" (Kaplan & Sadock, 1991) will help direct the nurse's interventions.

Health promotion usually involves changes in life style. These are difficult for people to make. Strategic interventions with patients can help them succeed in making changes.

Nurses often face dilemmas in patient care that involve noncompliance. Knowledge of legal precedents and standards should guide nurses' practice. In addition, nursing will be more effective if careful consideration has been given to thoughts and beliefs about conflictual situations. The best tools to deal with the challenge of noncompliance are self-awareness, a nursing philosophy grounded in mutuality, and excellent nursing assessment skills.

EXAM QUESTIONS

CHAPTER 11
Questions 73–78

73. What model postulates that patients choose noncompliant health actions on the basis of their perception that the illness is less of a problem than the treatment is?
    a. Health Belief Model
    b. Health Actions Model
    c. Predictors of Noncompliance Model
    d. Illness Perceptions Model

74. Which of the following is an environmental risk factor associated with noncompliance?
    a. Number of health care providers
    b. Limited income
    c. Credentials of care provider
    d. On-the-job support system

75. Which of the following is a characteristic of aging that affects noncompliance in the elderly?
    a. Fears about death
    b. Greater knowledge about disease in general
    c. Greater ability to think abstractly
    d. Greater numbers of prescribed medications

76. In dealing with noncompliance, what is the best tool the nurse has to affect a patient's behavior?
    a. Maturity
    b. Patience
    c. Self-awareness
    d. Caring attitude

77. The issue of mandatory drug testing is a good example of what ethical conflict?
    a. Rights of unborn fetuses versus rights of pregnant mothers
    b. The debate about the right to refuse treatment
    c. Rights of the individual versus the rights of society
    d. The debate about an individual's right to confidentiality

78. Which of the following is a defining characteristic of a competent patient?
    a. The patient has not been coerced into making a decision.
    b. The patient makes the right decisions for his or her health care situation.
    c. The patient is oriented and alert.
    d. The patient is physically and mentally able to participate in making decisions.

CHAPTER 12

NURSING MANAGEMENT OF THE MANIPULATIVE PATIENT

CHAPTER OBJECTIVE

After completing this chapter, the reader will be able to recognize manipulative behaviors and intervene appropriately.

LEARNING OBJECTIVES

After studying this chapter, the reader will be able to

1. Select the correct definition for manipulative behavior.

2. Distinguish between adaptive manipulation and maladaptive manipulation.

3. Recognize developmental patterns that may predispose the use of manipulation as a need-gratifying mechanism in adulthood.

4. Recognize the DSM-IV diagnoses that have manipulative behavior as a feature.

5. Specify criteria for nursing assessment of manipulative behavior.

6. Recognize the nursing diagnoses related to manipulative behavior.

7. Choose the most effective methods for intervening with manipulative patients.

DEFINITION OF TERMS

Manipulation is a method of interacting whereby a person attempts to gain control of others in order to fulfill his or her own needs and desires (Ellis, 1988). Webster's dictionary provides a succinct definition of the verb *manipulate:* "to control or play upon by artful, unfair, or insidious means, especially to one's own advantage; to change by artful or unfair means so as to serve one's own purpose."

The manipulator's goal is not only to get a particular need met but also to gain power over another person. As McMorrow (1981) put it, the manipulator "does not say 'please' to get a cookie, but to make the other person do as he wishes."

No other behavior in a patient evokes from nurses the singularly negative response that manipulativeness does. Try it. Tell another nurse a story about your most manipulative patient, and you are bound to elicit a groan of understanding. What is it about the manipulative patient that can turn a caring, understanding health care professional into an angry, withholding, frustrated one? And if manipulativeness evokes such a unanimously negative response, why does it seem that patients who use manipulation are so plentiful?

Adaptive Manipulation Versus Maladaptive Manipulation

Unquestionably, the word *manipulator* has

111

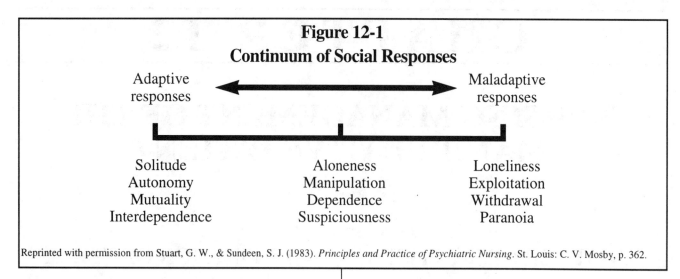

Figure 12-1
Continuum of Social Responses

Adaptive responses ← → Maladaptive responses

Solitude	Aloneness	Loneliness
Autonomy	Manipulation	Exploitation
Mutuality	Dependence	Withdrawal
Interdependence	Suspiciousness	Paranoia

Reprinted with permission from Stuart, G. W., & Sundeen, S. J. (1983). *Principles and Practice of Psychiatric Nursing.* St. Louis: C. V. Mosby, p. 362.

taken on a pejorative connotation. But the fact is that we all manipulate at times as a way of ensuring that our needs are met. Manipulation is a behavior that we learn to use early in life, and it is a process that occurs consciously or unconsciously in virtually all interpersonal interactions. In a healthy sense, manipulation refers to purposeful behavior aimed at getting one's needs met (McMorrow, 1981).

When manipulation is used in an adaptive sense, it is just one of a wide repertoire of behaviors that a person can call on to ensure that his or her needs are fulfilled. It is neither the only need-gratifying behavior nor the dominant one. Manipulation exists along a continuum of social responses *(Figure 12-1)*. The extent to which it is used as a dominant need-gratifying mechanism and the degree to which a person is aware of using it and of its effect on others partially determine whether manipulation is considered adaptive or maladaptive. It is important to understand that isolated uses of manipulation do not make a person a manipulator. The stress of hospitalization may cause a patient to resort to manipulation in an effort to meet needs that he or she is usually able to meet independently.

Illness poses a severe threat to security, self-esteem, and autonomy. It results in a loss of self-control and a fear of becoming helpless and dependent. The health care system often further strips patients of a sense of control. The resulting anxiety may prompt a regression to manipulation as a coping mechanism even in patients who are not typically manipulative. In the face of severe anxiety and a frightening awareness of their vulnerability, patients may attempt to manipulate the environment to regain a sense of self-control and self-mastery (Ellis, 1988). This anxiety-provoked regression may account for what is often perceived as an abundant use of manipulation among patients.

If everyone uses manipulation at one time or another, and if manipulation can be considered adaptive, how is the nurse to know when manipulation is constructive and when it is destructive? The following points help make the distinction (Wiley, 1968):

Adaptive, or constructive, manipulation

- Involves the use of a person's strengths and abilities to promote successful relationships.

- Is a conscious process on the part of both the manipulator and the person being manipulated. The manipulator takes responsibility for his or her behavior.

- Is mutually determined. Both parties in the interaction know what is occurring and can make a choice, on the basis on their own needs, as to whether to continue to participate in the situation.

Maladaptive, or destructive, manipulation

- Involves using others for one's own purposes. The manipulator promotes difficulties in or destroys relationships, and personal growth does not result.

- Is often unconscious. The person who is manipulated is unaware of the dynamics of the interaction and is aware only that he or she is experiencing negative feelings and is angry or wants to withdraw.

- Elicits further anxiety in the manipulator, whether or not his or her efforts are successful, and evokes an increased need to manipulate.

The Nurse-Patient Cycle of Manipulation

The manipulative patient—one who uses manipulation maladaptively—has little concern for the wants and needs of other people. Because manipulators do not trust their own feelings, they cannot trust others. This lack of trust leads to a sense of loss of control, and the manipulator tries to regain a sense of self-mastery by controlling others.

The manipulative patient is uncannily adept at seeking out others' unique weaknesses and vulnerabilities and using those weaknesses and vulnerabilities to gain control. Manipulative behavior can be active or passive (Chitty & Maynard, 1986). Active manipulation may involve any of the following behaviors:

- Making demands: "I want my medication at 9 o'clock, not 8 o'clock. I don't care about your rules!"

- Violating rules and routines: "Everyone has to be back from a day pass by 6 o'clock? Forget it! I'm going out with my friends. I'll get back when I'm good and ready."

- Making threats: "If you don't get that guy and his obnoxious family out of my room this minute, I'm going to tear up this place and you

along with it!"

Manipulative behaviors can also be passive, and far more subtle:

- Eliciting pity: "Can't you understand how hard it's been for me lately? My husband is leaving me for another woman, my two kids are out every night until 1 a.m., and my son wrecked a brand new car last weekend. Wouldn't you drink too?"

- Ingratiating and flattering: "You're the only one on this unit who can possibly understand me. I don't even know why you're working here—you're so much smarter than the rest of them. And prettier too."

- Evoking guilt feelings: "Well, if you had come in here to talk to me at 2:15, when you said you would, I wouldn't have gotten so depressed, and I wouldn't have had to cut my wrist."

- Abusing compassion: "You said you understood how hard it was for me to be in this hospital, so I was sure you'd understand why I needed to sneak out this morning. I'm back now, so take it easy. Why do you have to search me? You said you trusted me!"

- Attempting to exchange roles and become the helper's helper: "I heard you tell one of the nurses that you're having trouble with your son. I can't believe he doesn't appreciate having a mother like you. I'm about his age, I'll bet. Tell me what he's doing. Maybe I can help."

- Pitting staff members against each other: "I couldn't get that other nurse to understand why she should persuade the doctor to discharge me tomorrow. She said not to discuss it with you because you're too new to understand the rules yet. But I know you understand my situation. Will you explain it to my doctor? And pick a time when she's not around to interfere."

- Questioning competence or authority: "My

doctor said that I could have another sleeping pill if the first one didn't work. Can't you even read a chart? Well, you're not in charge around here anyway. We'll see what happens to your job when the nursing supervisor comes in tomorrow."

In each of the foregoing examples, the patient seized on a particular need of the nurse (the need to be professionally competent; to maintain a safe, consistent environment; to be viewed as empathic and understanding) and geared his or her behavior to exploit that Achilles' heel, that window of vulnerability.

Once a nurse realizes that he or she has been taken advantage of, has been successfully manipulated, his or her likely response is a range of negative feelings and behaviors, including anger, frustration, indifference, and withdrawal (McMorrow, 1981). Although the manipulative patient will enjoy these responses as signs of the patient's power, he or she will also feel an inward sense of increasing anxiety: Once again the patient has successfully managed to manipulate someone. Can no one be trusted? Will no one ever be able to see through the patient and give him or her what is truly needed—a sense of realistic limits and a genuine feeling of self-control? *Figure 12-2* illustrates the vicious circle of manipulation that can play out repeatedly between nurse and patient when manipulative behaviors are not accurately diagnosed and nursing interventions are not put in place to halt the cycle.

If the nurse is to act to stop the vicious circle, self-awareness is vital: The nurse with self-esteem needs is vulnerable to manipulative behavior (Chitty & Maynard, 1986). But who does not have such needs? The key is for the nurse to be aware of these needs so that she or he will know when they are being exploited. Nurses must be aware not only of their own vulnerabilities but also of their own responses—of their feelings of anger, need to withdraw, frustration, and loss of objectivity—as indicators that they are being manipulated. Only then can they be effective in helping the patient find more adaptive ways of getting his or her needs met.

A DEVELOPMENTAL VIEW OF MANIPULATION

Before nurses can intervene effectively, they must understand not only what manipulation is and how they respond to it but also where it begins. How does manipulation become entrenched as a need-gratifying mechanism?

The use of manipulation as an adaptive need-gratifying mechanism starts early in life. The term *adaptive maneuvering* has been coined to describe the manipulative responses of newborns (Kumler, 1963). Adaptive maneuvering is defined as an automatic behavioral pattern that a person adapts to decrease anxiety without learning or experiencing personal growth.

Newborns quickly and automatically learn several adaptive maneuvers to get their basic needs met. They manipulate without any regard for the needs of others. In newborns, who are utterly dependent on others, the use of manipulation is acceptable and, in fact, vital: It is a matter of survival.

As newborns grow and develop through childhood, they test a variety of adaptive maneuvers to manipulate the environment to gratify their needs. If a child's unacceptable experiments are met with clear and consistent limits delivered by primary caretakers with unconditional love and acceptance (of the child if not of the behavior), then the child will gradually develop a sense of self-esteem and self-control. Slowly, children learn to replace manipulation with more independent, adaptive behaviors. Above all, they learn to express their needs and to trust that those needs will be fulfilled (Ellis, 1988).

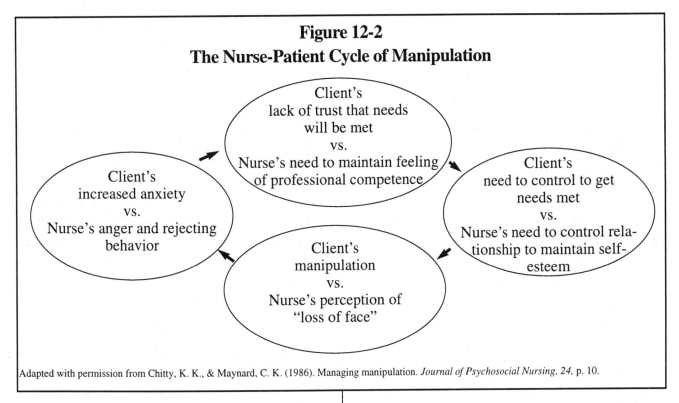

Figure 12-2
The Nurse-Patient Cycle of Manipulation

Client's lack of trust that needs will be met vs. Nurse's need to maintain feeling of professional competence

Client's increased anxiety vs. Nurse's anger and rejecting behavior

Client's need to control to get needs met vs. Nurse's need to control relationship to maintain self-esteem

Client's manipulation vs. Nurse's perception of "loss of face"

Adapted with permission from Chitty, K. K., & Maynard, C. K. (1986). Managing manipulation. *Journal of Psychosocial Nursing, 24,* p. 10.

If, on the other hand, a child's first limit-testing manipulative efforts are met with inconsistent limits or with no limits at all, with conditional love, and with lack of acceptance of the child, then the child will not learn how to fulfill his or her needs and how to gain love and acceptance from others. Because the child cannot trust that his or her needs will be met, he or she becomes profoundly anxious (Ellis, 1988; Stuart & Sundeen, 1990).

Thus begins the cycle of manipulation: A person has needs to be met but cannot trust the environment to meet them consistently. The ensuing anxiety causes the person to fall back on the earliest need-gratifying mechanism—adaptive maneuvering and manipulation—to ensure that his or her needs are met. If the manipulation is effective, the anxiety temporarily decreases. Success! The person's needs have been met. However, the pattern of manipulation has been reinforced. When the same person gets a negative response, he or she becomes angry and frustrated, and his or her anxiety skyrockets. The person again tries desperately to manipulate in an effort to regain control. The pattern is set.

Lacking basic trust, the person is caught in an endless cycle of having to manipulate in order to ensure that his or her needs are met—in order to survive. In the process, though, the person is likely to alienate all those around him or her, who soon learn that they cannot trust the person. The issue of developing trust, then, is key.

DSM-IV DIAGNOSES

As noted earlier, manipulation is ubiquitous. Nurses may encounter manipulation in any patient, on any unit, in any circumstance. However, some DSM-IV diagnoses are more likely than others to have manipulativeness as a characteristic:

- Conduct disorders
- Eating disorders
  Anorexia nervosa
  Bulimia nervosa
- Substances-related disorders
- Factitious disorders

- Personality disorders

    Histrionic personality disorder

    Narcissistic personality disorder

    Antisocial personality disorder

    Borderline personality disorder

    Dependent personality disorder

DSM-IV diagnoses provide good preliminary clues to manipulation. Any nurse assigned to a patient with one of the diagnoses in this list should be on the alert for manipulative behavior. However, it would be an error to rely on the DSM-IV diagnoses as a sole indicator. Many patients who have these diagnoses may not be maladaptively manipulative. The opposite is also true. Many patients who do not fit one of these diagnostic categories may use manipulation as a primary need-gratifying mechanism. Much more reliable then is a thorough nursing assessment.

NURSING ASSESSMENT: IDENTIFYING THE MANIPULATOR

The term manipulative, although a valid descriptor, may be overused by health care professionals. All nurses are prone, after a difficult day or after caring for a string of particularly taxing patients, to assign the label manipulator to the patient who makes that one final demand that sends them over the edge, or to the patient who is just a little too insistent in his or her self-advocacy. If the term manipulative is to have clinical meaning, its characteristics must be understood.

Manipulators are not always easy to recognize. They are often charming, entertaining, and intelligent. They rarely see themselves as having a problem and are unlikely to seek help on their own. In fact, many manipulators are loathe to change their behavior even when confronted with the reality of it, because it has inherent rewards. It gets their

needs met (Rawlins & Heacock, 1988). When the harmful effect on others is pointed out, the manipulator may feign guilt or remorse, because he or she is aware that these are the socially acceptable responses. But he or she will not actually feel these feelings. Manipulators do not have a superego strong enough for pangs of conscience to be genuine.

The reaction of the nurse faced with such a situation is, understandably, negative. This reaction is of more than casual interest, however. In fact, the nurse's feelings of anger and frustration constitute important clinical data that should not be ignored (Groves, 1978; McMorrow, 1981).

Murray and Huelskoetter (1983) cite the following warning signs of manipulation based on the nurse's feelings or subjective response to what is going on in the environment. They suggest that a manipulative patient may be at work when the following occur:

1. A previously harmonious staff is in an uproar over a treatment plan.

2. Patients are acting out and are being played against each other.

3. Family members are giving mixed and ambivalent messages about the patient.

4. Nurses feel that they are being bargained with or flattered.

Nursing diagnoses associated with manipulation most often have to do with powerlessness. Other nursing diagnoses include the following:

- Impaired social interaction

- Ineffective individual coping

- Disturbance in self-esteem

- Fear

- Risk for loneliness

PLANNING NURSING CARE

The next step toward intervening with the manipulative patient is to formulate long- and short-term goals. To ensure that every member of the staff carries out the treatment plan as consistently as possible—vital to ensuring that the patient cannot manipulate by "splitting" the staff—all team members should have input into setting goals. Certain goals should be considered in formulating the nursing care plan (Rawlins & Heacock, 1988).

The long-term goal is that the patient will determine and express needs and desires in a clear, direct manner that does no harm to others and that demonstrates responsibility for the patient's own actions.

The short-term goals are that the patient will do as follows:

- Recognize and verbalize feelings of anxiety, frustration, or powerlessness.

- Recognize instances of manipulative behavior.

- Gain insight into the effect of manipulative behavior on others.

- Distinguish between wants and needs and learn to delay immediate gratification of both.

- Verbalize acceptance of responsibility for own actions.

- Limit manipulative behavior and determine and practice alternative methods for gratifying needs.

NURSING INTERVENTIONS

Manipulative patients are a difficult nursing challenge. Although the nurse may be aware of a patient's manipulative coping mode, and the patient may be able and willing to recognize that pattern when it is pointed out, the patient may not be willing to change it. As noted previously, manipulation is inherently rewarding. However, manipulation also has a way of alienating others and of making it impossible for the patient to form meaningful relationships. The nurse who can help manipulative patients recognize the effects of their behavior and find alternative need-gratifying mechanisms will do much to improve the patients' quality of life. The following interventions may be useful:

- **Intervention:** Establish a trusting relationship.

  Rationale: Establishing a trusting relationship is as difficult as it is vital. Deception is a way of life for the manipulative patient, but every other intervention will be based on the foundation of a trusting nurse-patient relationship. It may be the first one that the patient has ever had in his or her life. Allow time for it to develop.

- **Intervention:** Recognize the problem and determine who generates it.

  Rationale: Patients cannot be helped to find more adaptive ways of living if they do not recognize their current behavior as a problem and if they cannot take some responsibility for the circumstances in which they find themselves.

- **Intervention:** Provide a consistent environment.

  Rationale: Inconsistent caretaking is at the root of the development of maladaptive manipulation as a coping mechanism in early childhood. The goal of manipulation is to somehow make the environment safe and secure. Knowing what to expect decreases the manipulative patient's anxiety and helps him or her learn to trust others and the environment. In addition, consistency reduces the patient's opportunity to divide the staff by manipulating them.

- **Intervention:** Refuse to respond to manipulation.

Rationale: Refusing to support the manipulative behavior tells manipulative patients that you cannot be used as an object. They will have to find another way of getting you to meet their needs.

- **Intervention:** Do not accept the behavior, but accept the patient.

Rationale: Manipulative patients are in desperate need of acceptance and positive regard. Try to get yourself—and the patient—to recognize the patient's behavior as manipulative rather than label the patient as a manipulator.

- **Intervention:** Help the patient to understand the impact of his or her behavior on others.

Rationale: Do not assume that empathy comes naturally to manipulative patients. Help them develop an awareness of their impact on others by being honest about your own feelings.

- **Intervention:** Set reasonable, clear, firm, consistent limits *(Table 12-1).*

Rationale: Although the patient will rail against them, he or she will be enormously relieved by them. They will provide the external control the patient needs until he or she can develop internal control.

- **Intervention:** Help the patient develop and practice alternative methods for gratifying needs.

Rationale: Manipulative patients will be loathe to give up a successful need-gratifying mechanism if they do not have another one with which to replace it.

- **Intervention:** Provide positive reinforcement every time the patient is able to communicate a need directly, take responsibility for himself or herself, or accept a limit.

Rationale: The patient needs to recognize not only unacceptable behavior but also acceptable behavior. Reinforcement of positive behavior is likely to elicit more positive behavior.

SUMMARY

The manipulative patient is among the most difficult of nursing challenges. Nurses may be well aware of the patient's desperate need for help and must get past a myriad of negative emotional responses of their own in order to give that help. Caring for these patients calls on all a nurse's skills as a practitioner and compassion as a human being: "Nurses who remember that control of behavior belongs to the client, not the staff, will be less likely to become enmeshed in power struggles...Listening and limit setting are nurses' most effective approaches for dealing with manipulation" (DeLaune, 1991).

Table 12-1
Ten Steps to Setting Limits with Manipulative Patients

1. Define clear expectations.

2. Communicate expectations positively and firmly.

3. Limit only those behaviors that clearly impinge on the well-being of the patient or others.

4. Make sure that the limits are in the patient's best interests and are not punitive.

5. Offer a brief rationale for the limit, but do not engage in a debate about its fairness or justification.

6. Define the consequences of exceeding the limit—and make sure that they are consequences that you can carry out.

7. Hold all discussions related to limit setting on a one-to-one basis, in private. (This limits the opportunity for the patient to involve an "audience" in determining whether the limit is "fair" or not.)

8. Make sure that all staff members understand the limit and its consequences as they were communicated to the patient.

9. Stand firm in the face of the inevitable testing of the limit.

10. Provide positive reinforcement each and every time the patient is able to meet the limit.

EXAM QUESTIONS

CHAPTER 12
Questions 79–85

79. Which of the following statements about manipulation is correct?

    a. It is always a sign of poor mental health.

    b. It develops during the turbulence of adolescence.

    c. It is always conscious.

    d. It is a behavior that everyone uses at one time or another.

80. Which of the following is true of maladaptive manipulation?

    a. It ends when the need is met.

    b. It is mutually determined by both parties.

    c. It leaves the person who was manipulated feeling angry but not necessarily certain about why.

    d. It can be growth producing.

81. At its most basic level, the development of manipulative behavior is a failure to do which of the following?

    a. Develop trust.

    b. Develop a sense of guilt.

    c. Develop love for one's caretakers.

    d. Experience anxiety.

82. According to the objective criteria for a nursing assessment of manipulation, which of the following scenarios describes a manipulative patient?

    a. At 10:45 a.m., for the second time, Mr. J. approaches the nurse's station for his 10:00 medications.

    b. The nurse observes Mr. B. hiding his medication under his pillow. He denies having done it and reminds her that he is the King of France.

    c. The nurse finds a bottle of whiskey in Ms. M.'s drawer. Ms. M. immediately admits to having hidden it there and is genuinely remorseful.

    d. Knowing that an important radiograph was scheduled for today, Mr. M. leaves the unit. He laughs when, on his return, the nurse reminds him that it is against policy to leave the hospital without informing the staff and that he missed a very important test.

83. Which of the following patients has met some important short-term goals for a manipulative patient?

    a. Ms. S. determines that the following are her three most important needs: a job, a place to live, and a new dress every week.

    b. Mr. J. admits that he broke the window in the patients' lounge but insists that it was not his fault; Mr. G. told him to do it.

    c. After calling a fellow patient a "worthless imbecile," Mr. R. is genuinely shocked to see her start to cry. He says he's sorry, but he has no idea what provoked her reaction.

    d. Mr. Y. approaches his primary nurse and discloses that he just told his student nurse that she was the only one who could understand his problem. He realizes that he was just trying to get some extra attention and asks the primary nurse whether she will spend 15 min with him in the afternoon.

84. The best care assignment for a manipulative patient who is expected to be on the unit for the next 3 weeks involves which of the following?

    a. Assigning a different nurse to the patient every day; this way no one gets "burned out."

    b. Assigning the same nurse to the patient every day and providing the nurse with plenty of peer support.

    c. Assigning "all staff" to take primary care of the patient; that way he'll get plenty of attention.

    d. Assigning as primary nurse the staff member who is leaving on vacation on Friday; he'll have time to recover.

85. Which of the following statements represents a well-set limit?

    a. Unit policy states that alcohol is not permitted in patients' rooms. Please get rid of that bottle now, or I will have to call security.

    b. You're always having too many people come up to visit you. No more visitors for the rest of the week.

    c. Everyone has to attend physical therapy. If you don't go, you can't have your medication at 2:00.

    d. Mr. A. brought a bottle of alcohol up to the unit, and that's against the unit's policy, so Mr. A. will not be permitted to have visitors for the rest of the week. Don't the rest of you think that's fair?

CHAPTER 13

NURSING MANAGEMENT OF THE PATIENT WITH CARDIOVASCULAR DISEASE

CHAPTER OBJECTIVE

After completing this chapter, the reader will be able to recognize common psychological responses to acute cardiac illness and those that occur in recovery phases.

LEARNING OBJECTIVES

After studying this chapter, the reader will be able to

1. Name at least two common responses to signs and symptoms of heart disease.

2. Differentiate between normal and abnormal psychological responses to acute cardiac illnesses.

3. State three characteristics of near-death experiences.

4. State two common family responses to acute illness of a family member.

5. Name three behaviors seen in patients in the recovery phase of cardiac illness.

6. Discuss nursing actions useful in the care of patients about to be transferred from the ICU.

INTRODUCTION

Persons at risk for coronary artery disease (CAD) share many common physiologic and psychosocial behavior traits. No one trait causes CAD, but the combination of traits increases the likelihood of the disease developing. Some traits cannot be changed, but most can be modified to decrease the risk of CAD. This chapter briefly reviews psychological risk factors. It goes beyond pre-CAD assessment to include common responses of patients and their families to critical cardiac illnesses and to the discharge and rehabilitation phases of CAD.

BEHAVIORS BEFORE THE ILLNESS

In addition to the physiologic risk factors for CAD, some psychological behaviors are common in persons in whom cardiac disease develops. Friedman and Rosenman (1974) have called these behaviors type A or coronary-prone behaviors. They contrast this behavior with type B behavior. In reality, few persons are purely type A or type B. Most have combinations of behavior styles but tend to lean one way or the other. Some behaviors are learned while the person is growing up; some develop later. None are so much a part of the personality that they cannot be changed. However, change can be difficult and requires a real commitment to be successful.

Type A behaviors typically occur in achievement-oriented persons who work with great intensity, aggression, and urgency to accomplish tasks. These people tend to struggle to fit more and more into less and less time. A type A person is always rushed, is impatient while waiting, and has difficulty letting others finish their thoughts or sentences. Type A persons expect others to share this intensity and to make the same commitments. The feeling of time urgency makes it difficult for type A persons to take time to be creative and leads them into stereotyped behavior in which they cannot accept change.

This achievement orientation is not limited to work; it extends into family relationships and the few outside activities that type A persons permit themselves. They may demand high achievement from their children in school or expect to be always on the winning team or to own the best car or home.

Any nurse who works with type A persons needs to understand their intense behavior patterns. Recognizing stress as a major risk factor of CAD is important. Telling patients to "decrease stress" will be futile. Patients must really believe that a stress reaction is harmful before they will attempt to change their behavior.

Patients who have chest pain during an intense business meeting may be able to correlate stress with heart disease. Patients may believe that they are at risk if others in their peer groups, who share the same life-styles, have heart attacks or must have cardiac surgery. Patients who have asymptomatic CAD will be the hardest to convince.

Patients who do relate their stress reactions to heart disease may have one or more responses. Those who perceive heart disease as a realistic threat to their lives may be motivated to make lifestyle changes.

Changes often are temporary because the patient reverts to a previous coping style. Denial of illness and total major restrictions in activity are opposing ways persons use to cope with a threat to their body image. A broken leg would slow down physical activity, but a diseased heart cannot be seen and therefore can be denied. Others are frightened by this threat, and they restrict all activity, becoming cardiac invalids.

Threats to self-image (the way a person sees himself or herself in relation to social and work roles) may make a person feel changed in an indescribable way. A patient may feel that he or she is no longer a competent provider or spouse, is not the same dynamic leader at work, or is useless and in the way.

BEHAVIORS DURING THE ACUTE ILLNESS

Shock and Disbelief

During the acute phase of cardiac illness, patients generally experience a normal grief response. The most common response to myocardial infarction is denial. Patients have a host of explanations for their signs and symptoms: indigestion, a pulled muscle, toothache, and so forth. They rationalize the manifestations by saying, "This cannot be happening to me. I just had a complete physical." Or, "I don't think my heart is the problem. Let me out of here."

It is important that lay persons be aware of this reaction and act quickly to obtain needed medical help. In the hospital setting, nurses need to know how the patient describes the symptoms: "pressure," "indigestion," "arm pain," or "chest pain." A patient who is experiencing intense substernal pressure may give a negative response to a question about chest pain and thus delay treatment.

While denying the severity of the illness, the patient also experiences fear, thinking, "What is happening to me," "Why can't I stop this pain," or "Am I dying?" This stage of shock and disbelief lasts a few minutes to a few days.

Development of Awareness

When patients realize that something is wrong

with their heart, they are becoming aware. In this stage, they move in and out of anger, bargaining, and depression. Anger may be directed at themselves or others, with comments such as "I did what my doctor said, but I still had a heart attack. What kind of doctor is he?" Or, "Why didn't I stop smoking earlier?" Or, "You don't let me sleep. No wonder I'm sick!"

Bargaining usually is done with a higher power or authority. It is not unusual to hear a patient say, "If I only live through this, I'll go to church regularly." Or, "If I get better, I'll stop smoking." Depression is common 3–5 days after a myocardial infarction. This is a time when the signs and symptoms usually have resolved, and the focus turns to what has happened to the patient and how it will affect the patient's life. Feelings of powerlessness and low self-esteem are common: "I can't do anything now. What good am I as a husband (or wife)?"

During the period of denial, it is important that the nurse allow this defense mechanism. Denial in the first hours and days of illness protects the patient from anxiety and fear. Anxiety and fear will increase the release of catecholamines, increase the myocardial workload of an already compromised heart, and thus promote further damage to the heart. Arguing with a patient in denial also increases the release of catecholamines and cardiac work.

Nursing actions need to support reality but not force it on the patient. Patients who will not believe that their heart is the problem and who want to be released from the ICU can be told, "I know it's hard to believe your heart could be the problem. Just to be sure, we need to keep you here for a few days to check blood tests and ECGs, which will give us the answer. How can I make your time here more comfortable?" Fear during this stage can be minimized with calm, truthful explanations and frequent bedside interactions. Sedative medications

may be useful also, but they never should be used in place of interpersonal communication.

As patients enter the period of developing awareness, the nurse will understand that their anger is not a personal attack but rather a way to release frustration and energy. Remember that many patients who have myocardial infarction are type A personalities who cope with stress by trying to get control over the situation and who are impatient with anything outside their usual activity schedules. Anger may be expressed in words or in actions (e.g., pulling off ECG leads, climbing over side rails, or refusing treatments).

The nurse should avoid arguing with the patient, but should set limits so patients will not harm themselves or others. Sometimes giving patients more control over their situation helps decrease anger and increase compliance. Letting the patient who is on bed rest sit in a chair may increase the patient's feeling of control, decrease anger, and consequently decrease the response of the sympathetic nervous system that otherwise would increase myocardial workload.

Bargaining may be done with a higher power, and patients may wish to see a clergy member. Bargains with physicians and nurses are usually long-term proposals (e.g., I'll quit smoking if I live through this) and need little intervention other than active listening. Short-term deals (e.g., I'll take my medicine if I can walk to the bathroom) should be addressed on a individual basis. A good approach is to do whatever will decrease the myocardial workload.

Depression is a source of concern to family members who now see the patient improving physically and cannot understand the patient's failure to feel positive. It is important to explain to both the patient and the patient's family that this is a normal stage of recovery. To help move patients through depression, increase their activity as soon as possible. Use a firm, kind approach to maintain the patient's self-respect as you get the patient up and bathed. Specific directions such as "walk to the next doorway and back three times each day" are more helpful than "gradually increase your activity." Depression that lasts longer than 1 week may require psychiatric intervention.

ICU Psychosis

ICU psychosis occurs to some extent in the majority of ICU patients within 2–5 days of their admission to the unit. Because the patients' usual behaviors and usual state of health are not known to the ICU staff, some of the subtle behavioral changes that precede the more obvious psychosis may be missed.

Characteristics of ICU psychosis are impaired intellectual function, difficulty in judging reality, and an altered emotional state in a high-stress situation. Behavioral manifestations may include the following:

- Having auditory and visual hallucinations (hearing and seeing things not present)

- Misinterpreting stimuli (e.g., confusion about health personnel in scrubs, who are interpreted as business persons inappropriately attired in pajamas)

- Talking with people not present (e.g., family, spirits)

- Having feelings of persecution, especially related to painful procedures (e.g., suctioning, insertion of IV lines, moving into a scanner for computed tomography)

- Pulling at tubes and wires and possibly doing self-harm

- Trying to get away from perceived danger by climbing out of bed

Factors that promote ICU psychosis include the following:

- Disturbed sleep cycles

- Absence of a day-night cycle

- Frequent contact with the many staff members for care

- Hearing staff members who are on rounds talk about the patients in the unit

- Proximity of other patients with their inherent odors, noises, and activities

- Multiple pieces of equipment within the line of vision

- Meaningless noises of machines

- Lack of usual sensory stimulation

- Sedation, which blurs consciousness

- History of psychiatric illness or of drug or alcohol abuse

- Prolonged cardiopulmonary bypass

Treatment of ICU psychosis. If admission to an ICU is anticipated (as occurs with patients who have cardiac surgery), preoperative teaching can help minimize the patient's confusion. Patients need to know that confusion and frightening dreams are common and do not indicate a psychiatric problem. They should be encouraged to discuss their fears before the operation and to share their feelings afterward.

Unplanned admission to the ICU adds another stressor for the patient. An accurate and thorough assessment is crucial, because differential diagnosis of psychosis is difficult. Additionally, up to 40% of patients with CAD have substance abuse problems that may result in a withdrawal syndrome during hospitalization.

To minimize ICU psychosis, decrease unnecessary stimuli. Turn off suctioning machinery when it is not in use. Move equipment out of the patient's line of vision. Turn off lights at night. Explain things that the patient does see and hear, including resuscitation efforts, insertion of IV lines, multiple infusion pumps, multiple personnel, and teaching rounds. Keep the patient oriented to the environment, ICU personnel, time, and current events. Explain all procedures before doing them. Be truthful about uncomfortable procedures so patients know that you do not mean to hurt them. Involve the family in the patient's care if they desire. Simple activities such as applying a cool cloth to the patient's head can be comforting to both the patient and the patient's family.

If ICU psychosis does occur, continue activities to minimize it. Be very simple and concrete in explanations. Do not agree with hallucinations, but do not belittle the patient. Statements such as the following do not take away the patient's self-respect, yet they promote orientation to reality: "I do not see those dogs that you see. I think they will go away as you get healthier." Support family members who may be frightened by the patient's bizarre behavior. Assure them that this is a temporary state and that it will pass.

Fortunately, ICU psychosis generally clears up after 24–48 hr on the regular nursing unit. Some confusion may take several days to resolve. Many patients do not remember any of the specific details of this period of time and need not be reminded. Patients' behaviors may be quite uncharacteristic and an unnecessary source of embarrassment for them.

Near-Death Experiences

The near-death experience is a psychological phenomenon of persons who come close to death. Some studies suggest that up to 50% persons who come close to death may have this experience. Many persons who have had a near-death experience are afraid to discuss it, thinking that they will be considered crazy. Others do not discuss it until many years after the experience.

Regardless of the person's age, sex, culture, religion, education, social class, or occupation, all near-death experiences have many things in common:

- Separation from the body occurs. Persons can relate what actually happened to them during the time they were out of their bodies, describe people never seen before or since, and tell how they felt as the health team worked to save their lives (some hoped not to be saved, and others hoped the resuscitation would be successful).

- Moving through a dark tunnel or space or through a fog is common. Many see a bright light on the other side that is associated with peace, love, and serenity.

- Many meet deceased relatives or friends, some of whom they may have had no knowledge of before the experience.

- Some meet a religious figure appropriate to their culture. This is not restricted to believers; it also occurs with nonbelievers.

- Persons see their lives pass before them or see significant people in their lives.

- Usually a sense of calm and relief from pain occur.

- Despite the pleasantness of the experience and the anticipation of pain on return, the persons understand a need to return to the body and do so.

- After the experience, persons have a sense of knowing about love and truth that they did not have before, and often they make life-style changes to promote this love.

Caring for a patient who has had a near-death experience requires sensitivity and patience. Even before you realize that a patient has had such an experience, you can help such patients by talking to them to keep them oriented about things going on during their unconscious period. Patients may be afraid to come right out and explain their experience for fear of being ridiculed. You can say that many persons who have been through a crisis like this have unusual experiences and leave an open-ended invitation for patients to talk about their own feelings.

It is important not to label near-death experiences as drug reactions or some psychopathologic response. Do not prod the patients; let them tell about their experience at their own pace. Reassure them that others have had similar experiences and refer them to support groups as needed (Corcoran, 1988).

Transfer Anxiety

A critically ill patient becomes dependent on the care of one or more nurses. Such patients are told that they are seriously ill, that they need total rest, that they need to let others take care of them. They are attached to several machines that monitor all bodily functions, and, despite the discomfort of wires, they become comfortable with the fact that any problems will be noted immediately and be taken care of. If the moment of transfer from the ICU comes suddenly, patients may be fearful that they are is being abandoned and that terrible things will happen to them. This type of anxiety also can occur as care is transferred from one nurse to another within the ICU setting.

Transfer out of the ICU should be treated as a graduation or promotion to be eagerly anticipated rather than a feeling of being dumped out for another patient's admission. In order to minimize transfer anxiety, it is important to prepare patients for the move. Show them how various monitoring devices are being removed as their health improves. Help them track their progress, for example, progressive ambulation, less IV medication to control chest pain, resolution of dysrhythmias, and healing of wounds. Give them progressively more responsibility for their care. For example, although a nurse could do the job more quickly, having patients bathe themselves gives them more independence and self-confidence.

Tell patients the expected length of stay in the ICU and where they will be cared for next. If possible, take them for a brief visit to the ward or step-down area before the transfer, or have the nurse from the ward see them in the ICU. At the time of transfer, introduce them to their new nurse (also applicable for shift-to-shift transfer within the ICU). This helps patients see that both nurses are part of the team and that care will be continued. If you promise to visit a patient after the transfer, keep your promise.

Sometimes patients are transferred suddenly because a more critical patient is admitted. This should be avoided if possible, because the patient may not feel ready. Keeping patients informed of their progress and of the plans for their transfer will help decrease the anxiety associated with sudden transfers. Coordination with physicians to transfer patients early enough to free beds for emergencies will help avoid the sudden transfer problem. If possible, visit suddenly transferred patients soon after the transfer to assure them of your interest in their welfare and of your coordination of their care with their new nurses.

HEART SURGERY

Deciding to Have Surgery

Deciding to have heart surgery is one of the biggest decisions many people make in a lifetime. The heart, the symbol of life, love, and courage, will be stopped, handled, cut, and sewn. No guarantee can be given that the operation will be successful or even that it will not be harmful. The patient looks forward to pain, prolonged recovery, financial expense, and possibly death.

Several factors can be helpful to the prospective patients and their families. Patients who see the surgery as giving them a new lease on life will approach the procedure positively. It is important that they do not view the operation as a cure for CAD or as a magic potion that will make them younger.

Patients need to be informed about complications, but they seem to focus more on life or death rather than the potential long-term complications (e.g., stroke, bleeding, infection, heart attack). Patients generally are more concerned about the reputation and skill of their surgeons than about the reputation of the hospital. After the procedure, they are more attuned to the fact that most postoperative care is provided by the nurse, not the surgeons. The patient who perceives that the benefits of surgery outweigh the risks probably will consent to have the procedure.

In one survey, patients were quite concerned with the need for psychological support. Several received no support from family physicians, cardiologists, or surgeons (Borders, 1985–1986). Nurses have a major role here. The nurse needs to have a strong knowledge base about CAD, available treatment options, and anticipated postoperative care and also needs to explore patients' feelings with them and with their families.

Patients may have preconceived ideas about heart surgery from the positive and negative experiences of friends, from popular magazines and television programs, from fellow patients, or from their own previous hospital experiences. They may have received medical information they did not understand. They may have unique concerns about family life, work, and finances.

Whenever possible, a group approach to preoperative teaching is useful to help patients share common concerns and develop a support group. Such an approach is also economical and time efficient for hospitals. Personal concerns then can be addressed on an individual basis.

Surviving Surgery

Waking up after surgery can be a confusing experience. The patient has lost a big block of time while anesthetized and awakens with tubes running in and out of every orifice in the body. Although patients may appear to be awake, it may take several more hours until they are fully awake. If they have had good preoperative instructions, a simple explanation of what is being done will usually set their minds at ease. If the surgery was emergency and no preoperative teaching was possible, the patient will need frequent explanations of care and restrictions.

Pain is usually a major postoperative concern. Many patients have no pain when lying still and only mild pain with activity. Others have significant pain while at rest and excruciating incisional chest pain with coughing and incisional leg pain with walking. The nurse should be aware of these variations in pain response and should give each patient adequate amounts of medication according to the patient's needs. The patient who is pain-free will be more relaxed and will cooperate more during treatments.

After the initial realization that they have survived surgery and have made it through 2 days of clinical progress, patients usually have a period of depression. This is similar to the depression seen in patients 3–4 days after a myocardial infarction. During this stage, patients cry easily, feel sicker, and have memory lapses. Patients who have been forewarned of this reaction usually have a less intense depression.

Going Home

Going home is a major milestone after heart surgery, but the joy is tempered by anxiety at leaving the security of the hospital. Spouses are also anxious because health care that was done by a professional team is being transferred to them. Like the transfer anxiety that occurs when moving from ICU to step-down or ward care, this anxiety can be minimized by good preparation, written instructions, and a telephone number to call for questions. Some hospitals have a nurse make a follow-up call to the patient's home the day after discharge to help ease the transition.

THE FAMILY'S RESPONSE TO CARDIAC ILLNESS

Families are an integral part of the patient and need to be considered when care is planned. The acute physiologic needs of the patient are always of prime importance. Ideally, the patient's nurse will be able to care for the family, too. However, many times the staffing demands of the unit do not provide for an extended time with patients' families. In this situation, a social worker or a member of the clergy may be designated for family support. This should not be left for whoever is available; it should be a designated assignment for some member of the health care team.

When patients are critically ill, they are usually isolated from their families for extended periods. Events may have evolved rapidly, leaving family members disoriented and afraid that their loved one may die. Depending on their life circumstances and usual coping behaviors, family members may feel anger at the patient or the health care team for the illness, guilt that they did not push the patient to treatment earlier, or depression and grief.

Family members react to these stressors in varied ways. They may minimize the illness to decrease the threat it imposes. Some intellectualize the illness by focusing on the technical aspects of care and blocking out emotional responses. Some repeat information received or the sequence of events as if to convince themselves of their appropriate response. One or more family members may be strong and supportive for other members. Many want to remain near the patient, either at the bedside or in a nearby waiting room (McGurn & Collins, 1981).

Nurses need to be aware of the family's needs. Nursing research studies have determined the needs of families of critically ill patients. Overall, the major one has been the need to have hope. The studies also have shown that often nurses did not rank family needs in the same order that the family did.

To most effectively care for the family, the nurse needs to take time to get to know family members, their past experiences, and their needs as individuals. They should be encouraged to talk with the nurse, social worker, or clergy as well as among themselves. Verbalizing fears and needs is usually more helpful than keeping silent about them. Provide privacy during brief family visits in the ICU. Encourage hugs, kisses, or other signs of affection if desired. Make yourself available to a designated family member who calls to get a report on the patient's condition. Convey all messages to the patient. This kind of tie to the family at home can be therapeutic.

Once the critical illness is over and the patient is moved out of the ICU, families may be forgotten. Without frequent updates and progress reports, family members imagine all sorts of complications occurring. Keep patients and their families aware of progress to decrease unnecessary anxiety and to prepare a smooth transition to discharge from the hospital.

Homecoming for any cardiac patient may be met with a variety of emotions. The spouse may harbor suppressed anger at the patient for being ill, out of work, and shirking duties. The spouse may feel guilty if the illness occurred during sexual relations or when the patient was doing work for the spouse. Spouses often overprotect the patient, both as an expression of love and concern and out of fear that something will go wrong. Open communication in the hospital and at home is the key to minimizing homecoming anxiety.

RECOVERY BEHAVIORS

Recovery is a prolonged period that begins with discharge from the hospital and lasts for the rest of the patient's life. Patients may expect to return immediately to their previous level of activity, but find that they are weak, anxious, and depressed. They may have trouble sleeping because of a fear of dying. They may feel stifled by overprotection of their spouse, yet be afraid to be home alone. If they perceive their health as poor, they will have a slow return to normal life.

Family conflicts occur because of changes needed in diet, activity, and medications. Some patients may not be able to return to previous jobs or to any work. Spouses and other family members may have assumed new roles in the patient's absence. Well-intentioned attempts to take over responsibilities and free the patient from pressures actually may diminish the patient's self-esteem and promote family conflict.

The nurse can prepare the patient and family for this recovery period by comprehensive teaching started several days before the patient's discharge. The patient and the patient's spouse should be present so they hear the same instructions and can ask questions. A group class is helpful for patients with similar problems so that families can learn from one another.

Patients and families need to know about anticipated emotional responses and to plan how they will handle these responses without hurting others. Instructions on diet, activity, and medications should be given. Spouses need to understand the instructions, but they should not nag the competent patients to follow the instructions. Creating the situation at home so that discharge procedures can be followed and giving the patient the choice of following them puts the responsibility where it belongs, with the competent adult patient, and will minimize family conflict. Follow-up medical care also needs to be discussed.

Rehabilitation is a lifelong process. It is easier for patients to stay motivated if they have family and group support. Cooking prudent heart-healthy meals for the whole family increases compliance more than making one meal for the patient and another meal for the others. Exercise as a part of the daily routine and done with one or more per-

sons is more successful than walking alone while others stay in bed.

Formal groups for patients (e.g., Mended Hearts) and spouses are helpful for sharing concerns and for problem solving. The American Heart Association and the patient's hospital staff can suggest groups that meet patients' and families' needs. A family physician who maintains close contact with the patient gives assurance of an interest in the patient's welfare and increases the patient's compliance.

SUMMARY

Psychological care of cardiac patients is a vital part of their recovery from illness. The heart symbolizes life, love, and emotions. Injury to the heart cuts to the very core of life and leaves patients and their families afraid of death or of radically changed lives. Comprehensive nursing care from the acute illness through recovery will help modify the psychological stress of cardiac illness and will promote full recovery for patients and their families.

EXAM QUESTIONS

CHAPTER 13
Questions 86–90

86. A type A person has just been told by a physician to cut back work hours to help decrease stress-induced hypertension How would this person most likely respond?

    a. I've been noticing a lot of pressure at work, and I planned to cut back.

    b. I'm busy working on a big project. I need to work more hours, not fewer.

    c. You're probably right. I'll give my biggest account to my partner to finish.

    d. I'll just take a little nap after lunch and that will help with my stress.

87. Your patient says, "You don't know what you are doing! No wonder I'm not getting well faster!" What stage of grief is this patient in?

    a. Bargaining

    b. Denial

    c. Anger

    d. Depression

88. Which of the following is true about patients' reactions to the diagnosis of myocardial infarction?

    a. Denial is a protective mechanism in the first hours after diagnosis.

    b. Anger is a childlike response and should be punished.

    c. Nonbelievers will not try bargaining because they do not believe in a higher power.

    d. Most patients accept the diagnosis quickly because the physician tells them it is true.

89. Which of the following might help minimize patients' anxiety at the time of transfer from the ICU to the ward?

    a. Keep them informed of their progress and the anticipated date of transfer.

    b. Sympathize with them about the lack of good care on the wards.

    c. Do not talk about the transfer until it is happening so that you do not get their hopes up.

    d. Tell them you will keep them in the ICU as long as possible so that they will be safe.

90. Patients who are discharged from the hospital after cardiac surgery or treatment for cardiovascular disease usually feel which of the following?

    a. Ready to get back to work as soon as possible

    b. Glad to turn over their usual responsibilities to other family members

    c. A renewed strength to get up and entertain visitors

    d. Frightened, anxious, and, possibly, depressed

CHAPTER 14

USE AND ADMINISTRATION OF PSYCHOTROPIC MEDICATIONS

CHAPTER OBJECTIVE

After completing this chapter, the reader will be able to specify the classifications of psychotropic medications and indicate the applicable nursing principles for the administration of these drugs.

LEARNING OBJECTIVES

After studying this chapter, the reader will be able to

1. Recognize which medications are antipsychotics, anxiolytics, antidepressants, and mood stabilizers.

2. Recognize the signs and symptoms that may be relieved by each of these classes of psychotropic medications.

3. Specify the potential side effects associated with the use of psychotropic medications.

OVERVIEW

Psychotropic medications are used throughout the general hospital. They are prescribed for both long- and short-term use and are highly effective in treating the intended signs and symptoms.

Some patients who are taking psychotropic medications may need to have the drugs discontinued temporarily (e.g., for surgery). Administration should begin again when medically appropriate and ordered. Additionally, the nurse should be particularly observant for changes in the patient's mood and behavior to assess the effectiveness of the medications.

Some patients may be just beginning a course of a psychotropic medication (e.g., an antidepressant) while in the hospital primarily or secondarily for the treatment of depression. Others may be taking a psychotropic medication on an ongoing basis and be hospitalized for an unrelated condition (e.g., hypertension). In administering the medication, the nurse should be prepared to teach the patient important information about the drug's action and potential side effects.

ANTIPSYCHOTICS

Antipsychotic medications (*Table 14-1*) are sometimes referred to as neuroleptics or major tranquilizers. Although they may have some uncomfortable side effects, they generally are considered safe and quite effective in decreasing some of the major signs and symptoms of psychosis, such as hallucinations, delusions, anxiety, and agitation.

Antipsychotics help stabilize a person's thoughts, behaviors, and moods. They do not cure schizophrenia, but they are generally effective in the treatment of altered thought processes. The

Table 14-1
Antipsychotics

Generic Name	Trade Name	Adult Oral Maintenance Dose Range (mg/day)
Chlorpromazine	Thorazine	30–900
Thioridazine	Mellaril	20–200
Trifluoperazine	Stelazine	15–20
Perphenazine	Trilafon	12–64
Acetophenazine maleate	Tindal	60–120
Prochlorperazine	Compazine	15–150
Fluphenazine	Prolixin	1–5
Chlorprothixene	Taractan	75–600
Thiothixene	Navane	20–30
Haloperidol	Haldol	1–15
Loxapine succinate	Loxitane	30–100
Clozapine	Clozaril	300–600
Mesoridazine	Serentil	30–150
Risperidone	Risperdal	4–6

Source: Spratto, G. R., & Woods, A. L. (1995). *Nurse's drug reference 95.* Albany, NY: Delmar Publishing.

drugs help a psychotic patient feel more normal and thereby better able to function. Antipsychotics may make some patients who have schizophrenia more able to interact in psychotherapeutic treatment.

Uses

In an acute care setting, antipsychotic medications may be used to treat psychoses that are part of an organic mental disorder, which may occur because of a disease or because of the toxic effects of some chemical, medication, or treatment.

Anxiety disorders can be treated beneficially with antipsychotics (consider the amount of psychological stress that occurs in an acute illness), although the minor tranquilizers would be the first-line drugs of choice. The side effect of tranquilization is helpful for patients who are anxious.

Psychotic and agitated depressions may be seen in an acute care setting, although they are sometimes mistaken for something else, such as a physical symptom or an organic illness. Antipsychotics can be useful in these situations.

The signs and symptoms that may respond to antipsychotics include the following:

- Hallucinations
- Delusions
- Paranoia
- Anxiety and agitation
- Hostility and rage
- Aggression and assaultiveness
- Flight of ideas, loose associations, illogical thinking
- Sleep disturbances

Nonpsychological signs and symptoms that are sometimes treated with antipsychotics include nausea and vomiting and intractable hiccoughs.

Antipsychotic medications may be used for

prolonged periods, even years, either continuously or sporadically. These drugs are helpful in relieving some of the clinical manifestations of the following disorders:

- Schizophrenia
- Thought disorders
- Bipolar affective disorders
- Affective disorders
- Anxiety disorders

Action

Although different chemical groups are involved, it is widely believed that the antipsychotics work by blocking the neurotransmitter dopamine at the postsynaptic neuron receptor sites throughout the brain. This mechanism of action is effective for controlling target symptoms, but it also causes the extrapyramidal side effects that are so discomforting for some patients.

The major classes of antipsychotics are as follows:

- Phenothiazines
- Aliphatics
- Piperidines
- Piperazines
- Thioxanthenes
- Butyrophenones
- Dihydroindolones
- Dibenzoazapines
- Diphenyl-butylpiperidines

The potency of antipsychotics may be high or low. The highly potent medications such as Haldol (haloperidol) and Prolixin (fluphenazine) have a greater antipsychotic effect per milligram; thus smaller doses are used. Highly potent antipsychotics are the least sedating, and the prevalence of extrapyramidal side effects is high. On the other hand, higher doses of the lower potency medications such as Thorazine (chlorpromazine) and

Trilafon (perphenazine) are required to produce an antipsychotic effect. These medications are more sedating, but the prevalence of extrapyramidal side effects is lower.

Since the early 1990s, newer antipsychotic medications have appeared on the market that offer effective treatment in many cases in which the older antipsychotic medications did not work. The newer drugs include Clozaril (clozapine) and Risperdal (risperidone). These new antipsychotics offer hope to many people with chronic thought disorders, whose symptoms have been refractive to previous treatments. Agranulocytosis is a common side effect of Clozaril, so patients taking this medication require weekly monitoring of their white blood cell count.

General Properties

The antipsychotics are considered fairly safe, even in high doses for some. They are nonaddicting and produce no euphoria or tolerance. These are not drugs of abuse. It can take several hours to as long as weeks before the maximum antipsychotic effect occurs, and full improvement may not be reached until later still.

Some antipsychotics are injectable. Others are available as tablets, capsules, or liquid concentrates. Haldol Decanoate and Prolixin Decanoate are available in long-acting forms; injections are given every 1–4 weeks.

Choosing the right drug for each patient requires consideration of multiple factors. These might include a patient's response in the past, the response of a blood-related family member, the manifestation of the illness, and the medication's side effects (beneficial or deleterious).

Side Effects

The more common side effects of antipsychotic medications are usually not dangerous or severe, although the rarer side effects can be so severe as to be life-threatening. The ramifications of neuroleptic malignancy syndrome or tardive dyskinesia cannot be discounted. Many of the more minor side effects are quite irritating, but accommodation usually occurs after a few weeks, and some side effects are diminished completely.

Antipsychotics differ in the severity and type of side effects they commonly produce. Each drug should be reviewed for its specific potential side effects before it is administered.

Some of the side effects may appear to be an increase in the signs and symptoms of the psychosis rather than a side effect (e.g., akathesia). Nurses who are knowledgeable about the signs and symptoms of both the disease and the potential side effects of these drugs do their patients a great service by managing drug-induced problems at the earliest onset.

Extrapyramidal side effects. Extrapyramidal side effects are common with antispychotics. Pseudo-parkinsonian syndrome, which resembles Parkinson's disease, may develop. The signs and symptoms include a masklike face, shuffling gait, and tremors. Excessive drooling and muscle rigidity may occur.

Akathesia is a feeling of motor restlessness; the legs will not stay still. The patient may have an uncomfortable feeling of internal agitation or restlessness. Patients who experience akathesia may become noncompliant in taking their medications. This symptom is quite troublesome to patients, but it usually can be treated successfully with Cogentin (benztropine mesylate) or Benadryl (diphenhydramine hydrochloride).

Dyskinesias are involuntary movements that seem coordinated and have a rhythmic pattern. They usually involve the arms, legs, and trunk. Dystonias are also involuntary movements. They are more jerky than dyskinesias. The movements are uncoordinated and spastic, and they have no pattern. Sometimes the patient appears to be locked, fixed, or stuck in an uncomfortable posi-

tion. The neck and face are affected in torticollis, the torso and back in opisthotonos, and the eyes in oculogyric crisis. Dystonic reactions are a true emergency and need immediate treatment, usually an injection of Cogentin or Benadryl.

Tardive dyskinesia is one of the more serious and prolonged of the extrapyramidal side effects. If early signs of tardive dyskinesia are detected (through an Abnormal Involuntary Movement Scale), it is prudent to discontinue the current medication regimen. When high doses of antipsychotics are used, this side effect occasionally has an early onset. In other cases, the onset may be later, perhaps after many years of use and after a cessation of the medication. This side effect is sometimes irreversible if not detected early. Currently, no definitive treatment is available for tardive dyskinesia, although much research is being conducted to discover effective remedies for this syndrome.

Patients who have tardive dyskinesia experience involuntary rhythmic movements of the mouth that include sucking, chewing, licking, and pursing movements. The tongue may protrude, and the face may be affected (e.g., rapid eye blinking). A rockinglike movement of the whole body also may occur.

Other side effects. Many side effects other than the extrapyramidal ones are associated with the use of antipsychotics. The following is a partial description of some of the more common ones.

Drowsiness is one side effect that can be beneficial, and it should be considered when determining the right medication for someone. Drowsiness may be desired or may be purposefully avoided. For a patient who has been agitated, restless, and sleepless, this side effect will be beneficial. For one who has had difficulty functioning or is fatigued and tired, perhaps oversleeping or staying in bed, drowsiness as a side effect to be avoided.

Anticholinergic side effects generally include

dry mouth, blurred vision, constipation, and nasal congestion. Patients commonly complain of these and often become accommodated to them. Urinary problems such as hesitancy or, more seriously, retention also can occur.

Orthostatic hypotension may occur, and patients may become accommodated to it. However, although this side effect is acute, the patient may experience fainting episodes and periods of light-headedness. Patients should be cautioned to rise slowly from a lying to a sitting position before standing. The patient's blood pressure should be monitored regularly.

Skin reactions may occur. A rash is seen sometimes on the trunk and back. Patients can become photosensitive and thus need protection when out of doors. The liquid-concentrate form of Thorazine can cause a contact dermatitis, perhaps to the nurse who administers this medication. Endocrine changes may be induced. Menstrual malfunctions such as amenorrhea may occur, galactorrhea is seen occasionally, and some men may have gynecomastia. Sexual functioning and desire may be changed and limited.

Occasionally seen are seizures, abdominal distress, weight gain, jaundice, retinopathy, hyperglycemia, and cardiac changes. Not often seen but potentially lethal are agranulocytosis and neuroleptic malignant syndrome.

Agranulocytosis is a severe decrease in the number of white blood cells. Early signs and symptoms are sore throat, high fever, and mouth sores. Neuroleptic malignant syndrome is an idiosyncratic problem generally seen with the high-potency, long-acting medications, such as Prolixin. The syndrome is similar to malignant hyperthermia. The patient has a change in consciousness, autonomic instability, moderate-to-high fever, and severe rigidity.

Without treatment, neuroleptic malignant syndrome progresses rapidly; a decline in the patient's condition occurs within 12–24 hr. Because the signs and symptoms are generally insidious, the syndrome sometimes is not detected, and patients are thought to be having a worsening of their psychosis. An increase in the serum level of creatinine phosphokinase is one of the early confirmatory clinical indicators. Neuroleptic malignant syndrome is clearly a life-threatening medical emergency, necessitating an ICU setting for monitoring and treatment.

Relief of signs and symptoms. As noted previously, the more common side effects of antipsychotic medications are generally effectively treated. Antiparkinsonian medications and antihistamines may produce acute relief of signs and symptoms for some problems associated with the use of antipsychotics. Benadryl and Cogentin are widely used to reverse the discomforting problems of extrapyramidal side effects.

Dietary changes may help with gastrointestinal and weight problems. Chewing gum or sucking candies is helpful for a dry mouth. Keeping busy and well occupied provides some relief in some cases. Stress reduction can be helpful when patients are preoccupied with some signs or symptoms. Physical exercise also can produce some relief.

Contraindications

Some preexisting medical problems may require the complete cessation or avoidance of an antipsychotic. Consideration should be given to the severity of the psychosis and the potential harm that may occur because of it (the traditional risk vs. benefit analysis). The following conditions should be considered before treatment with antipsychotics is started:

- CNS depression
- Blood dyscrasias
- Pregnancy and lactation
- Benign prostatic hypertrophy

- Previous allergic response
- Kidney and liver problems
- Glaucoma

ANXIOLYTICS

The anxiolytic drugs *(Table 14-2)* are effective in producing a calming effect, a tranquil effect, and sleep. Many of these medications are potentially drugs of abuse and misuse. However, the benefits to some patients are notable, and general hospital nurses can expect to see these drugs widely prescribed. Short-term use of these medications is the best method for preventing abuse or addiction.

In addition to producing calming and relief from anxiety, high stress, and panic, the anxiolytics, also called minor tranquilizers, commonly are used in withdrawal regimens from alcohol and some addictions in which the drugs are cross-tolerant, particularly Librium or Ativan. Anxiolytics may also be ordered for sleep, for muscle tension, and for either chronic or acute anxiety states.

In general, anxiolytics are safe. However, tolerance and addiction do occur over time. The daytime sedation effect must be monitored in active and fully functioning persons. Patients who use these drugs for a long time will go through withdrawal when the drug is stopped or the dosage is decreased. Such withdrawal may happen inadvertently in the general hospital if patients who are taking these medicines at home do not let the staff know at the time of admission. These patients may become delirious, have severe episodes of anxiety and restlessness, have intense insomnia, or experience seizures. This possibility reinforces the need to obtain thorough drug histories from all patients. Instead of taking these medicines on an ongoing basis, it may be more productive for the patient to take them periodically for an acute problem and then discontinue them.

Uses

The main mode of action of anxiolytics is depression of the CNS. Their uses in clinical practice include the following:

- Promotion of sleep and sedation
- Relief from or lessening of anxiety
- Detoxification in treatment of drug addiction (Librium or Ativan)
- Muscle relaxation (Valium)
- Preoperative and postoperative sedation

Side Effects

The most common side effects associated with the use of anxiolytics include the following:

- Tolerance and addiction
- Daytime sedation and clouding of consciousness
- Impaired judgment
- Paradoxical agitation

The elderly seem to be particularly prone to some of these side effects, even though these medications often are prescribed for this age group.

Contraindications

Anxiolytics should be prescribed with caution for the following:

- Known drug addicts, unless used in the medical management of a withdrawal regimen
- Patients with a compromised respiratory system
- Patients with severe liver damage
- Women who are pregnant or breast-feeding

ANTIDEPRESSANTS

Antidepressant medications *(Table 14-3)* are another category of commonly used psychotropic medications that, along with the antipsychotics and anxiolytics, may be seen in the general hospital. They are generally grouped

Table 14-2
Anxiolytics

Generic Name	Trade Name	Adult Oral Dose (mg/day)
Alprazolam	Xanax	0.75–4
Buspirone HCl	BuSpar	15–60
Chlordiazepoxide HCl	Librium	15–100
Clorazepate dipotassium	Tranxene	15–60
Diazepam	Valium	4–40
Halazepam	Paxipam	60–120
Hydroxyzine HCl	Atarax, Vistaril	200–400
Lorazepam	Ativan	2–6
Meprobamate	Equanil, Miltown	1200–2400
Oxazepam	Serax	30–120

Source: Spratto, G. R., & Woods, A. L. (1995). *Nurse's drug reference 95.* Albany, NY: Delmar Publishing.

into three major types: tricyclic antidepressants (TCAs), monoamine oxidase inhibitors (MAOIs), and selective serotonin reuptake inhibitors (SSRIs). Although other antidepressants (e.g., the tetracyclics) are available, these three types are the most widely used. Antidepressants are effective in alleviating signs and symptoms of depression in 70–80% of cases.

Tricyclic Antidepressants

Although still a topic of research, the biochemical genesis of depression is fairly well accepted, partly because of the successful clinical results seen with the use of antidepressants. There seems to be a correlation between depression and the neurotransmitters norepinephrine and serotonin. These biochemicals are stored in nerve cells and promote impulse transmission.

When more neurotransmitters are available at the postsynaptic cleft, the signs and symptoms of depression seem to be fewer. Tricyclic and related antidepressants seem to increase the availability of neurotransmitters by preventing the reuptake of these biochemicals into the nerve cells. The neurotransmitters are not removed and so their concentrations within the synapse remain higher.

Tricyclic antidepressants have been in clinical use since the mid-1950s. Amitriptyline and imipramine (Elavil and Tofranil) have been used as a mainstay of antidepressant treatment for more than 30 years.

Use. Tricyclic antidepressants are marketed specifically for the treatment of depression. They have different side effects, which may be more beneficial or harmful in different people. For example, some may cause drowsiness and thus would be a good choice for a depressed person who has insomnia.

It is not easily known in advance which patient will respond to which of the TCAs, although a history (family or individual) of effective treatment with one TCA favors the use of that drug. Otherwise, a trial-and-error approach can be used (time permitting) if the patient's signs and symptoms are not too devastating and do not cause marked dysfunction. A specific antidepressant may be chosen because of an associated side effect or avoided because of a specific contraindication.

Researchers are investigating which drugs

affect norepinephrine levels and which ones affect serotonin levels and the correlation with the signs and symptoms of depression that different people have. The hope is that we will be able to predict accurately which medication will be the best one for each particular patient.

Patients often have more than one psychiatric disorder or illness. It is not unusual for someone who has chemical dependence problems, an eating disorder, or a personality disorder to have depression also or to respond to an antidepressant as part of their treatment regimen even thought they have no clear-cut signs and symptoms of depression.

The drug imipramine is used in severe cases of enuresis in young children. A TCA introduced in 1989, clomipramine, has shown good results in patients with obsessive-compulsive disorders. With some exceptions, the TCAs generally require 2–3 weeks of continuous use before beneficial results are seen. Patients should be educated about this so they do not expect relief prematurely and thus think that they are not getting better, which can be discouraging.

Case example. A 60-year-old woman was markedly depressed after cardiac surgery. Her physician prescribed a low dose of amitriptyline for her to take each night and described the medication as an antidepressant that would bring her relief. The patient began taking the medication at home but found herself becoming more and more unhappy. She awakened each night at 2 a.m.; she had no appetite; and although she had been encouraged to take short walks, she found herself too tired. She began sobbing uncontrollably and felt internally agitated. After only 4 days on the medication, she attempted to commit suicide by taking an overdose of sleeping pills and left a note, which read, "I am such a failure, even the antidepressant couldn't cure me. I might as well end my life now and no longer be a burden to anyone."

This patient surely would have benefited from the knowledge of how long it takes before an antidepressant results in symptomatic relief.

Side effects. The specific side effects of TCAs vary somewhat from drug to drug and from person to person. The most common complaints and problems are the following:

- Dry mouth
- Blurred vision
- Constipation
- Urinary retention
- Orthostatic hypotension
- Tachycardia and palpitations
- Sleep problems: insomnia or drowsiness
- Ataxia, unsteadiness, and tremulousness
- Weight gain or loss
- Paradoxical confusion, mania, or psychosis

Contraindications. Tricyclic antidepressants must be used cautiously in patients who have cardiac conditions. A complete physical assessment and medical clearance should be obtained. Potential problems also should be considered in patients who have the following:

- Glaucoma, narrow angle
- Urinary problems, retention
- Benign prostatic hypertrophy
- Seizure disorders
- Impaired liver function

Caution: During the early stages of therapy with TCAs, suicidal tendencies can increase as the depression lifts and the patient now has the energy to kill himself or herself. These drugs are a potent means with which to overdose. Close supervision by staff is imperative at this time.

Monoamine Oxidase Inhibitors

Monoamine oxidase is an enzyme that metabolizes the neurotransmitters, and MAOIs prevent this metabolization. The result is an increase in the

Table 14-3
Antidepressants

Generic Name	Trade Name	Adult Oral Dose (mg/day)
Tricyclics		
Amitriptyline HCl	Elavil	75–150
Nortriptyline HCl	Aventyl, Pamelor	75–150
Protriptyline HCl	Vivactil	15–60
Imipramine HCl	Tofranil	75–300
Desipramine HCl	Norpramin	50–300
Trimipramine maleate	Surmontil	75–200
Doxepin HCl	Sinequan, Adapin	75–200
Clomipramine	Anafranil	100–250
Maprotiline HCl	Ludiomil	75–225
Amoxapine	Asendin	150–300
Monoamine Oxidase Inhibitors		
Isocarboxazid	Marplan	10–30
Phenelzine sulfate	Nardil	45–60
Tranylcypromine sulfate	Parnate	20–30
Selective Serotonin Reuptake Inhibitors		
Paroxetine HCl	Paxil	20–50
Vanlafaxine HCl	Effexor	75–225
Sertraline HCl	Zoloft	50–200
Fluoxetine HCl	Prozac	20–80
Others		
Trazodone HCl	Desyrel	150–400
Bupropion HCl	Wellbutrin	300–450

Source: *Nursing 93 drug handbook.* (1993). Springhouse, PA: Springhouse Corp.; and Spratto, G. R., & Woods, A. L. (1995). *Nurse's drug reference 95.* Albany, NY: Delmar Publishing.

amount of neurotransmitters available for neuronal activity.

These medications also have a long history of use with depression. For some time now, MAOIs have been less popular because of the required dietary restrictions. Some patients, however, do well while taking these drugs and manage with little or no side effects or major sequelae. The antidepressant effect of an MAOI can seem quite remarkable for some patients with severe depres- sions for whom the TCAs are ineffective. Monoamine oxidase inhibitors are also effective in the management of panic disorder and phobic disorders.

Monoamine oxidase inhibitors are strong anti- depressants that require particular attention to the dietary restriction of tyramine. Ingestion of foods containing tyramine can precipitate an acute hyper- tensive crisis. This dietary restriction has prevented MAOIs from being as popular as the TCAs and the newer antidepressants. For this reason, MAOIs are rarely used as first-line drugs for the treatment of depression.

Use. The MAOIs are used in the treatment of depression. A tyramine-free diet must be followed to avoid the danger of a hypertensive crisis. Some of the foods to be avoided include the following:

- Aged cheese

- Red wine

- Beer

- Chocolate

- Yeast products

- Yogurt

- Pickled products

- Soy sauce

Additionally, some medications can cause the same problem. These include Ritalin (methylphenidate), Demerol (meperidine), and most of the over-the-counter cold and diet preparations. Nurses who care for patients who are taking MAOIs should review with the patients a complete list of foods and medications to be avoided. As well, MAOIs and TCAs should not be given together, except under rare, closely monitored situations.

Side effects. Possible side effects associated with the use of MAOIs include the following:

- Dry mouth

- Constipation

- Blurred vision

- Orthostatic hypotension

- Urinary problems

- Edema

- Confusion

Contraindications. Use of MAOIs should be avoided in patients who are considered unreliable or who cannot maintain the dietary restrictions. Patients should be assessed medically, and use of

these antidepressants avoided if there is evidence of the following:

- Liver and kidney disease

- Hypertension

- Hyperthyroidism

- Seizure disorders

- Pheochromocytoma

- Glaucoma

Selective Serotonin Reuptake Inhibitors

The SSRIs exploded onto the market in the late 1980s with the introduction of Prozac (fluoxetine) for the treatment of depression. This drug, as well as its successors, is highly effective in the treatment of depression.

Relief from the signs and symptoms of depression generally occurs after 3–5 days of use, compared with 10–14 days for the TCAs. An additional benefit is the milder side effects. Like the TCAs, the SSRIs can cause a manic episode. Therefore, patients taking these inhibitors should be monitored for any changes in behavior. Another potential side effect is acute aggressive reaction, which could necessitate discontinuance of the medication.

Lithium Carbonate

Lithium carbonate, a mood stabilizer, is used primarily as the drug of choice in the treatment of bipolar affective illness. It often is started during the manic phase of the disorder. Patients who have been stabilized successfully with lithium may need to take it long term. The anticonvulsant Tegretol (carbamazepine) has also been used as a mood stabilizer, for patients who are refractive to lithium therapy or are bothered by the side effects of lithium.

Lithium is a simple cation, like sodium and potassium. A specific concentration of lithium in the blood must be maintained to produce stabilization of a patient's signs and symptoms. The specific mechanism of action for lithium carbonate and exactly how it works in stabilizing the highs and lows of bipolar affective illness are unknown. Even so, its effects are sometimes dramatic and remarkable. The behavior and thought processes of manic patients can change markedly once lithium therapy is started. After taking this medication for 7 days, patients may have a dramatic improvement in their manic behavior.

The dose range of lithium has a narrow margin of safety. Blood levels of the drug must be monitored by analyzing blood samples obtained 8–12 hr after the patient's last dose of lithium. The frequency of monitoring can be decreased as use of lithium progresses from initial titration to long-term maintenance. Initially, blood levels may be monitored two or more times each week. After a patient has been stabilized, one time each month may be adequate.

Serum levels of lithium of 0.5–1.2 mEq/L are generally considered safe and effective. Levels greater than 1.5 mEq/L suggest apparent or potential lithium poisoning. The usual daily dose of lithium is 300–1800 mg. The dosage might be 900–1200 mg taken as 300 mg three or four times.

Aside from dose of medication, there is a cause-and-effect relationship between lithium and sodium and fluid balance. Lithium and sodium affect the fluid balance in the body.

Patients who are taking lithium must maintain an adequate intake of fluids and salt. A decrease in the intake of either or both of these increases the potential for lithium retention, which will cause the serum level of lithium to rise. Alternatively, if the intake of sodium or fluids or both is an increased, the amount of lithium excreted increases, causing a decrease in the serum level of lithium. Patients should follow their physician's advice if they are on a low-salt diet, take diuretics, change their intake of sodium or fluids, or perspire a lot. All these can affect the serum level of lithium.

Lithium poisoning can be fatal. Poisoning is progressive and can be detected early by monitoring the early signs and symptoms of toxic effects and by measuring the levels of lithium. Some of the early signs and symptoms of toxic effects include the following:

- Fainting
- Lethargy and sluggishness
- Slurred speech
- Nausea, vomiting, and diarrhea
- Thirst, dry mouth, bloated stomach
- Tremors, especially of the hands
- Ataxia
- Anorexia

The more pronounced signs include the following:

- Muscle fasciculations
- Seizures
- Change in consciousness
- Electrolyte imbalance
- Cardiac problems

Side effects. Lithium has side effects that are commonly seen in many patients and sometimes jeopardize the patients' compliance with lithium therapy. These include the following:

- Nausea
- Vomiting
- Diarrhea
- Excessive urination
- Abdominal cramping
- Hand tremors
- Muscle weakness, stiffness
- Fatigue, sluggishness
- Weight gain
- Metallic taste in the mouth

In addition, an impairment in kidney or thyroid functioning, which is usually reversible, may occur with long-term use. Patients on long-term lithium therapy should have a complete physical examination every 6 months, including a check of kidney and thyroid functioning.

Contraindications. Patients should have a physical examination before lithium therapy is started. The drug should be used cautiously in patients who have the following:

- Cardiac problems
- Myasthenia gravis
- Organic brain syndrome
- Seizure disorders
- Parkinson's disease
- Pregnancy (also women who are lactating)
- Kidney problems
- Thyroid disorders

As with many potent medications, the potential benefits must be weighed against the potential risks. This list is not complete, and each patient's physical condition should be considered before treatment with lithium is begun.

NURSING INTERVENTIONS

The role of the nurse in the administration of psychotropic medications is consistent with administration of all medications given to a patient by a nurse.

Patients who need a psychotropic medication have been experiencing some problem with their emotions, cognition, or behavior. As with communication and interpersonal skills, the administration of these medications sometimes requires special consideration.

The following interventions can be used for patients who are taking a psychotropic medication:

- Assess the patient and review the patient's history for contraindications.
- Monitor the patient's vital signs.
- Administer the medication as prescribed.
- Observe for potential side effects.
- Educate the patient and the patient's family about the medication.
- Observe for evidence of the medication's effectiveness in alleviating the target symptoms.

EXAM QUESTIONS

CHAPTER 14
Questions 91–96

91. Which of the following are antipsychotic medications?

    a. Thorazine and Haldol

    b. Mellaril and Elavil

    c. Elavil and Tofranil

    d. Valium and Librium

92. Antipsychotics are used to treat which of the following?

    a. Toxic reactions and hiccoughs

    b. Delusions and hallucinations

    c. Depression

    d. Extrapyramidal side effects

93. Which of the following are both anxiolytics?

    a. Clonazepam and Clozaril

    b. Temazepam and diazepam

    c. Haldol and amobarbital

    d. Xanax and Valium

94. Which of the following is a toxic serum level of lithium?

    a. 0.02 mEq/L

    b. 1.20 mEq/L

    c. 0.25 mEq/L

    d. 2.50 mEq/L

95. Addiction is a potential danger associated with use of which of the following drugs?

    a. Antipsychotics

    b. Haldol

    c. Lithium carbonate

    d. Anxiolytics

96. Which of the following are antidepressants?

    a. Prozac, trazodone

    b. Halcion, Haldol

    c. Desyrel, diazepam

    d. Elavil, Mellaril

CHAPTER 15

ETHICAL AND LEGAL ISSUES IN PSYCHIATRIC NURSING

CHAPTER OBJECTIVE

After completing this chapter, the reader will be able to recognize the ethical and legal issues that are of concern in the practice of psychiatric and mental health nursing.

LEARNING OBJECTIVES

After studying this chapter, the reader will be able to

1. Specify the basic ethical issues cited by Bandman and Bandman.

2. Recognize the provisions in the American Nurses Association (ANA) Code for Nurses.

3. Specify the standards of practice for psychiatric and mental nursing established by the ANA.

4. Recognize current issues in the ethical and legal aspects of nursing practice.

OVERVIEW

All areas and specialties of nursing are affected by issues of ethics and matters pertaining to the legal aspects of health care. Ethical and legal issues go hand in hand.

Ethical issues are those involving decisions whereby a moral judgment comes into play. Ethics in nursing practice are concerned with doing good for patients while avoiding doing any harm to them

(Bandman & Bandman, 1990).

The legal issues in nursing practice are those matters that not only require a moral judgment but also are mandated by the justice system. In dealing with these issues, nurses are held accountable, and therefore punishable, by law.

ETHICAL ISSUES

Bandman and Bandman cite five ethical issues, some of which seem clear and some of which may be controversial, that pertain to the practice of general nursing.

1. Quality of life versus quantity of life

2. Freedom versus control and prevention from harm

3. Telling a truth versus telling a lie

4. Desire for knowledge versus religious, political, economic and ideological interests

5. Conventional, scientific-based therapy versus alternative, nonscientific types of therapy and treatment

Code for Nurses

The ANA has a code for nurses (ANA, 1985) that offers guidelines for nursing practice. The specific provisions of this code are as follows:

1. The nurse provides services with respect for human dignity and the uniqueness of the client unrestricted by considerations of social or eco-

nomic status, personal attributes, or the nature of health problems.

2. The nurse safeguards the client's right to privacy by judiciously protecting information of a confidential nature.

3. The nurse acts to safeguard the client and the public when health care and safety are affected by the incompetent, unethical, or illegal practice of any person.

4. The nurse assumes responsibility and accountability for individual nursing judgments and actions.

5. The nurse maintains competence in nursing.

6. The nurse exercises informed judgment and uses individual competence and qualifications as criteria in seeking consultation, accepting responsibilities, and delegating nursing activities to others.

7. The nurse participates in activities that contribute to the ongoing development of the profession's body of knowledge.

8. The nurse participates in the profession's efforts to implement and improve standards of nursing.

9. The nurse participates in the profession's efforts to establish and maintain conditions of employment conducive to high-quality nursing care.

10. The nurse participates in the profession's effort to protect the public from misinformation and misrepresentation and to maintain the integrity of nursing.

11. The nurse collaborates with members of the health professions and other citizens in promoting community and national efforts to meet the health needs of the public.

Standards of Practice for Psychiatric Nurses

The ANA also provides standards of practice for different specialty groups within the nursing profession. The following are taken from the ANA's *Standards of Psychiatric and Mental Health Nursing Practice* (1994). Items 1–6 concern practice standards of psychiatric and mental health nurses; items 7–11 concern performance standards of the same specialty.

1. The nurse collects client health data.

2. The nurse analyzes the assessment data in determining diagnoses.

3. The nurse determines expected outcomes individualized to the client.

4. The nurse develops a plan of care that prescribes interventions to attain expected outcomes.

5. The nurse implements the interventions specified in the plan of care.

- The nurse uses counseling interventions to assist clients in improving or regaining their previous coping abilities, fostering mental health, and preventing mental illness and disability.

- The nurse provides, structures, and maintains a therapeutic environment in collaboration with the client and other health care providers.

- The nurse structures interventions around the client's activities of daily living to foster self-care and mental and physical well-being.

- The nurse uses knowledge of psychobiological interventions and applies clinical skills to restore the client's health and prevent further disability.

- The nurse, through health teaching, assists clients in achieving satisfying, productive, and healthy patterns of living.

- The nurse provides case management to coordinate comprehensive health services and ensure continuity of care.

- The nurse uses strategies and interventions

to promote and maintain mental health and prevent mental illness.

6. The nurse evaluates the client's progress in attaining expected outcomes.

7. The nurse systematically evaluates the quality of care and effectiveness of psychiatric and mental health nursing practice.

8. The nurse evaluates his or her own psychiatric and mental health nursing practice in relation to professional practice standards and relevant statutes and regulations.

9. The nurse acquires and maintains current knowledge in nursing practice.

10. The nurse contributes to the professional development of peers, colleagues, and others.

11. The nurse's decisions and actions on behalf of clients are determined in an ethical manner.

Nurses who work with psychiatric patients or deal with psychosocial issues in the general hospital follow many of these standards, and all nurses in any field should be guided by the Code for Nurses.

LEGAL ISSUES

The legal aspects of health care delivery services and practitioners are guided by criminal law, as are all persons by virtue of being members of society. In addition, mental health laws give further guidance in situations that include persons who may be harmful to themselves or others or are judged unable to care for themselves because they are significantly disabled because of a mental illness.

Least Restrictive Alternative

The concept of least restrictive alternative stems from a legal decision made in the case of *Rouse v. Cameron* in 1966. It was ruled that the court could no longer order a patient to be "hospitalized" involuntarily if reasonable alternative treatment plans could be offered. The court noted that the purpose of involuntary hospitalization is treatment [and concluded that] the absence of treatment draws into question the constitutionality of the confinement (Kaplan & Sadock, 1991).

Therefore, if treatment is not a part of the involuntary hospitalization, the patient may participate in a therapeutic program through an outpatient clinic, day hospital, residential treatment center, or group home. Patients will benefit most from this arrangement if they have sufficient social, family, and community supports to use these means as an adjunct to individual or group and family counseling.

The state can insist on treating a patient. In the best interests of the mentally ill who cannot care for themselves, each state does have the right to provide sufficient care and treatment, but it must offer this in the least restrictive manner available.

This issue has ethical concerns as well as legal ramifications. Those who believe in absolute rights for all persons, despite handicaps or inabilities, take issue with the paternalistic power the government is exhibiting in the role of caretaker or surrogate parent to someone who is mentally ill. "Human rights vs. human needs creates a struggle between the legal and psychiatric professions for dominance over the conceptualization and management controls of the mentally ill" (Garritson, 1983). In his book *The Myth of Mental Illness,* Thomas Szasz argues that the various psychiatric diagnoses are totally devoid of significance and contends that psychiatrists have no place in the courts of law and that all forced confinements because of mental illness are unjust (Kaplan & Sadock, 1991).

Involuntary Hospitalization

The courts continue to determine the need for involuntary hospitalization for persons who are considered to be a danger to themselves or others or who are so incapacitated by their mental illness that they cannot care for themselves. The ethical questions continue and will thus keep the issue of individual liberty alive.

Whereas the concept of the least restrictive alternative is applied to degree and means of treatment, the involuntary hospitalization of someone pertains to a most basic right. The Constitution of the United States guarantees all persons the right to pursue liberty. When the court orders involuntary hospitalization of someone who has not committed a crime, it is depriving that person of his or her basic right to be free.

The alternative point of view focuses on the mentally ill person who is considered to pose a clear and present danger to himself or herself or others, someone who is suicidal or homicidal and refuses treatment. In these instances, the government has the right to hospitalize that person involuntarily on a temporary basis. Additionally, it is the responsibility of the state to maintain the welfare of the public and keep it free from potential harm as may sometimes be the case.

Procedures, which are similar from state to state, delineate the process of involuntary hospitalization as practiced in each jurisdiction. The rights of the mentally ill person are protected by the inclusion of the following:

- Notification of when and why a commitment procedure will be held

- A specified amount of time, which may differ from state to state, for which someone may be held against his or her will pending a formal hearing (varies from 72 hr to perhaps as long as 2 weeks)

- Representation by an attorney and access to this legal counsel in an unobstructive manner

- Some clear and convincing proof of dangerousness or inability to function (The Supreme Court ruled on this issue in 1979, in the case of *Addington v. Texas.*)

Involuntary hospitalization because of a court order is for a specified period. At the end of that period, the patient is entitled to an additional hearing if there is further need or disagreement on the need for continued hospitalization. Although most states rely on physicians to participate in the process of involuntary hospitalization, some recognize nurses as being qualified to certify the need for this action (Laben & MacLean, 1989). Although general hospital nurses usually are not involved in the process, psychiatric nurses should be aware of their own state mandates.

The moral and ethical concerns stemming from the 1960s policy of deinstitutionalization has become apparent with the increase in need and ability to hospitalize persons against their will. The idea of releasing mentally ill patients from public institutions that were large, sometimes isolated, and in shocking states of disarray and bedlam, seemed noble at the time. Unfortunately, the unacceptably low number of public community outreach programs to assist these mentally ill individuals has caused deinstitutionalization to fail.

There is some public outcry, seemingly associated with the increased number of homeless persons, many of whom are mentally ill. Unless a change occurs in the trend of decreasing funding to support the infrastructure needed for the deinstitutionalized population, deinstitutionalization will remain a failed public policy (Kaplan & Sadock, 1991).

Right to Refuse Treatment

The past 40 years have seen the increasing use of psychotropic medications in the treatment of the mentally ill. Although these medications may produce some remarkable and dramatic changes in a patient's aberrant behavior, they are not without their own side effects, and some patients may not want to take them. This issue of a patient's right to refuse medication has posed controversies in some cases, such as patients who are hospitalized involuntarily.

The case of *Rennie v. Klein* (1983) addressed the right of an involuntary patient to refuse treatment. The court ruled "on the basis of the right to privacy that mentally ill patients in nonemergency situations could refuse treatment. However, it is a qualified right, taking into account the patient's threat of physical harm to other persons, the patient's capacity to make decisions for himself [or herself], the existence and availability of less restrictive treatment and the risk of permanent side effects" (Laben & Maclean, 1989). In addition to the right to refuse psychotropic medications, the right to refuse treatment may pertain to the use of involuntary seclusion and mechanical restraint.

Informed Consent

Tied to the issue of the patient's right to refuse treatment is the issue of informed consent. To agree to or refuse treatment, the patient must be aware of what the proposed treatment includes, the reasons for it, the possible dangers, and any alternatives available. "Informed consent is the cornerstone of autonomy theory. Adult patients are assumed to have the right to consent to or refuse to consent to treatment" (Kaplan & Sadock, 1991).

Informed consent is an issue throughout the general hospital and in general nursing practice. "Regarding medical, surgical or diagnostic procedures, a patient has the right to his [or her] diagnosis, prognosis, and the risks, benefits, and alternatives to the proposed measures in words the patient can understand" (Bandman & Bandman, 1990).

Which member of the health care team is designated to obtain informed consent should be clearly understood by all concerned and should be indicated in the hospital's policy and procedure manual. Usually informed consent for operative and other invasive procedures falls in the domain of the physician. Review of the informed consent may fall to the nurse, and if the nurse thinks the patient does not adequately understand the procedure, the nurse must notify the physician.

In addition to providing information about medical procedures, "nurses should become acutely aware of the importance of providing information to clients about nursing procedures. If a client has questions pertaining to the procedure or to administration of medication, answers should be given as clearly and succinctly as possible. The client should be involved in the decision making about procedures and the taking of medication. The nurse must be willing to clarify information and discuss questions on an ongoing basis. If queries arise concerning a medical procedure, the physician should be notified. It should also be noted that the client can revoke consent for a treatment or procedure at any time" (Laben & Maclean, 1989).

Competency

Competence is determined on the basis of a person's ability to make a sound judgment (Kaplan & Sadock, 1991). The opportunity to give informed consent is expected to be made available to persons who are presumed to be competent. "There is a popular misconception that an involuntarily hospitalized patient is assumed incompetent. Actually, the law presumes every adult to be competent even if committed to a mental health facility" (Snyder, 1984). Legally, someone is not considered incompetent until a court declares him or her to be so.

In most instances, persons who have reached the age of 18 are permitted to manage their own property and health in any manner that they desire. Although a person may be functionally unable to make appropriate decisions regarding his or her health or finances, that person is still considered legally competent until a court declares the person incompetent and appoints a guardian or conservator to act on his or her behalf as guardian of his or her person or estate or both (Laben & MacLean, 1989).

Patients' Rights

When patients are institutionalized, their rights as patients are preserved according to the guidelines of the particular institution they are in. The rights of all patients in general hospitals are guided by the American Hospital Association's *A Patient's Bill of Rights* (1992). This bill defines the following rights of patients:

- The patient has the right to considerate and respectful care.

- The patient has the right to and is encouraged to obtain from physicians and other direct caregivers relevant, current, and understandable information about diagnosis, treatment, and prognosis.

- The patient has the right to make decisions about the plan of care before and during the course of treatment and to refuse a recommended treatment or plan of care to the extent permitted by law and to be informed of the medical consequences of this action.

- The patient has the right to have an advance directive concerning treatment or designating a surrogate decision maker with the expectation that the hospital will honor the intent of that directive to the extent permitted by law and hospital policy.

- The patient has the right to every consideration of privacy.

- The patient has the right to expect that all communications and records pertaining to his or her care will be treated as confidential by the hospital, except in cases such as suspected abuse and public health hazards, when reporting is permitted or required by law.

- The patient has a right to review the records pertaining to his or her medical care and to have the information explained or interpreted as necessary, except when restricted by law.

- The patient has the right to expect that, within its capacity and policies, a hospital will make an appropriate and reasonable response to the request of a patient for appropriate and medically indicated care and services.

- The patient has the right to ask about and be informed of the existence of business relationships among the hospital, educational institutions, other health care providers, or payers that may influence the patient's treatment and care.

- The patient has the right to consent to or decline to participate in proposed research studies or human experimentation that affect care and treatment or require direct involvement of patients and to have those studies fully explained before the patient gives consent.

- The patient has the right to expect reasonable continuity of care when appropriate and to be informed by physicians and other caregivers of available and realistic care options when hospital care is no longer appropriate.

- The patient has the right to be informed of hospital policies and practices that relate to patients' care, treatment, and responsibilities.

Confidentiality and Privilege

Understanding the issues of confidentiality and privilege is imperative when providing therapeutic care to patients. Confidentiality is the legal and ethical responsibility to keep all information about patients private. Nurses as well as other health professionals must not divulge or release information given or available to them as part of their professional duties to persons not properly authorized access to that information (Laben & Maclean, 1989).

Privilege is a narrower concept: "the right to maintain secrecy or confidentiality in the face of a subpoena." This right belongs to the patient (Kaplan & Sadock, 1991). It is created by state statute to protect information received from clients and is granted only to specific professionals to ensure that the information will be kept private and confidential unless the client waives the privilege. The issues of confidentiality and privilege, although always an important right of an individual, carry an additional importance when related to a psychiatric patient, because of the nature of the information involved.

Duty to Warn

Relevant to working with the mentally ill is the 1976 decision in the case of *Tarasoff v. Regents of the University of California.* This case mandated that when a patient threatens to harm another individual, therapists have the duty to warn the individual, the individual's family or friends, or the authorities and thus have the duty to exercise reasonable care to protect the foreseeable victim of danger (Laben & MacLean, 1989).

NURSING IMPLICATIONS

These areas of ethical and legal concerns need to be examined carefully. When in doubt about the nursing implications, nurses should consult with the other members of the health team and their own supervisors for guidelines.

It is important to maintain confidential relationships with patients. Nurses should establish whether or not the statutory privilege has been enacted by the legislature in their state and whether or not it includes nursing privilege (Laben & MacLean, 1989).

The legal and ethical issues of general hospital nursing and those specifically pertaining to psychiatric nursing interrelate when a nurse is working with a patient on a general hospital unit who may be mentally ill. It is an important part of nursing practice to maintain an awareness of the current issues.

CASE STUDIES

Chemical Dependency

Marvin Collins is a 49-year-old man who works as a commodities trader and part-time real estate broker. Mr. Collins was admitted, through the emergency department, to a cardiac unit to have his status monitored after an episode of crushing chest pain with evidence of valve collapse. He was awaiting test results on his cardiac status to determine his need and suitability for bypass surgery.

On his first day on the unit, he appeared tense, nervous, and jittery. Although anxiety would be an appropriate response in his situation, the agitation seemed more than appropriate to the situation, according to Margarette Ray, Mr. Collins's primary nurse.

Ms. Ray noticed that the patient was anxious, diaphoretic, tremulous, and sleepless. He had a rapid pulse, high blood pressure, an elevated body temperature, and loss of appetite. Although some of these signs and symptoms were attributable to his cardiac condition and his concern about it, Mr. Collins seemed to be in additional distress.

Margarette Ray had 15 years of experience as a nurse. She planned her morning to include 10 min to sit and talk with Mr. Collins. She did not have the time to do a formal mental status examination, but she followed her intuition and asked the patient about his alcohol intake.

Mr. Collins admitted to excessive drinking. He not only drank a fifth of vodka every two nights but also drank every day at lunch, had two to three martinis each day, and had some bloody Marys 3–4 days a week "to get the day going right." He talked of feeling tremulous without drinking and said that by having a nip early in the day, he could keep up his pace.

Understanding that Ms. Ray was concerned with his consumption, Mr. Collins quickly added,

"At least I'm not snorting the white stuff through my nose like my coworkers. What can be harmful about drinking? I've always been a drinker; I can hold my liquor!"

Mr. Collins did need bypass surgery. He was transferred to a cardiac surgery unit. Ms. Ray made sure to include his drinking history in his transfer report. Now in his third hospitalized day, Mr. Collins was at great risk for alcohol withdrawal. His surgery was successful, with a brief stay on a cardiac postoperative unit and then a transfer back to his original unit.

Ms. Ray was Mr. Collins's nurse once again. She followed up by discussing his previous drinking behavior with him; this discussion was an important aspect of his discharge planning. She then conferred with his cardiologist, Dr. Cook. Although Mr. Collins had not as yet experienced terribly negative effects from his alcoholism, the serious and fragile nature of his medical condition precluded his ability to return to the same patterns and habits. In addition, his present drinking pattern most likely would soon get him into deeper trouble with alcoholism.

As part of the discharge planning, Dr. Cook recommended that Mr. Collins participate in AA meetings. This participation would help Mr. Collins come to terms with his drinking problem. Although Mr. Collins protested that he did not have a problem, Dr. Cook stood firm in the recommendation and presented other outpatient options, a local chemical dependency program he knew of and therapy with a psychiatrist colleague who worked in addiction medicine.

During Mr. Collins's cardiac rehabilitation on the cardiac unit, Ms. Ray, who had established a rapport with him, helped him open up to her a little bit. She reviewed with him the dynamics and causes of his drinking behavior and the effect this behavior had on his general health and well-being.

This case is a typical example of a patient who is admitted to a general hospital with a primary disease or disorder that requires some medical or surgical intervention. In this situation, the patient's nurse can act as a primary resource in assessing health problems and then can collaborate with the patient and other health care providers to provide interventions to treat the secondary or underlying problem. Often seen, alcohol and other substance abuse problems can be addressed first by a nurse in this manner.

The Suicidal Patient

A 26-year-old woman was brought by ambulance to the emergency department of a large medical center. A neighbor had found the patient moaning and lying on the floor of the patient's apartment just inside the door. The patient's left hand had been almost severed.

The patient's name was Andrea Jarrod. It was learned that she had a history of paranoid schizophrenia and depression. Although she was in shock and not communicative, it appeared to the neighbor and the ambulance attendants that she had cut her own wrist with a meat cleaver.

The ambulance attendants had carefully packed the partially severed hand in saline, wrapping it well and keeping it close to the patient's arm. She was admitted directly to the operating room, where a microsurgery team was quickly gathered to perform the procedures that ultimately took 14 hr to reattach her hand.

After the surgery, the patient was taken to the recovery room, where she awoke in a few hours. Her vital signs were stabilizing, and her left arm was elevated, held up to an IV pole by a complicated pulley system of gauze wrap. The surgery was considered successful. The hand was fully reattached, and within a few days it would be clearer how much return of functioning could be expected.

The recovery room nurse, Deborah Miller, knew that until this time, Ms. Jarrod had not spoken with anyone. The nurse was concerned that on awakening the patient would still be suicidal. While the patient slept, the usual routine of one nurse for two patients seemed sufficient. Once the patient was awake, Ms. Miller instituted the following psychosocial nursing care measures, with were done in the recovery room:

- A mental status examination was performed when the patient was awake and was alert.

- A lethality assessment was made of the patient's current suicidal ideation.

- Constant observation was initiated. A nursing aide would stay with the patient at all times. In order to be effective, this meant within arm's length and always within eye view. If the aide needed relief, direct switch of staff members was done; the patient was never alone.

- A bedside search was done. Potentially dangerous objects were removed. The usual bedside treatment setup (e.g., instruments, wound cleanser) was removed after each use.

- The patient's family was notified. Her parents, who lived in another state, made plans to visit immediately.

- The patient's therapist, a clinical nurse specialist, was notified, as was the psychiatrist the patient had been seeing for medication therapy.

Although Ms. Jarrod said that she did not feel suicidal, the severity of her initial attempt was so great that until her therapist arrived, it was thought best for the staff to maintain the one-to-one constant watch.

Ms. Jarrod was transferred to a surgical unit. The nurses there already had been apprised of the situation, one that is generally uncomfortable for general hospital nurses. The patient's primary nurse on the surgical unit, Dede August, already was working out a plan that would follow the guidelines of the recovery room staff.

The patient was put in a private room next to the nurses' station and within eye view of it. The room was assessed for potential danger. Sharp objects and cleaning agents were removed. The staff agreed not to keep treatment materials at the bedside. The patient's chart was clearly marked: SUICIDAL PRECAUTIONS.

Communications with the patient made it clear that she was psychotic and quite paranoid. Although she remained quiet, when asked she clearly described voices that she heard telling her "bad things": "They told me to cut off my arm so I would be forgiven. The poisons needed a way to drain out." When not communicating, she was observed to be apparently hallucinating; she was attentive to something and was seen talking animatedly to no one present.

Constant observation was continued by the staff. As staffing permitted, each nurse and aide was assigned a 30- to 60-min block of time to be with the patient. The stimuli in this busy surgical room were decreased as much as possible. Antipsychotic and antidepressant medications were started.

Ms. August called a patient care conference with all the team members present. Together they formulated a care plan that all would consistently follow. All staff members were informed that this patient needed to be witnessed swallowing her medications, so there would be no opportunity for her to cheek her medications and save them up for a possible future overdose.

Ms. August carefully documented the care plan and ensuing events in the patient's chart, making sure to put in specific things the patient had said so that all staff members would understand what was meant by hallucinations, paranoid ideation, and suicidal ideation.

The care plan included designating a period of 30 min each shift to be spent sitting at the patient's bedside to encourage verbalization. Ms. August made an attempt to begin a trusting relationship with the patient. The nurse was supportive and reassuring. When some new or painful procedure needed to be done, she tried to be there.

Reality testing and reorientation were done. Ms. August tried to monitor the severity of the patient's psychosis and to report the same, noting any changes from the previous day or days. At least once each shift, the patient was asked about her suicidal ideation and an assessment was made of her mental status.

After 8 days on the postsurgical unit, the patient's condition had stabilized enough so she could be transferred to a locked inpatient unit in the psychiatric clinic attached to the hospital. Ms. August continued to visit every 2 or 3 days, at the encouragement of the psychiatric staff and the patient, who had begun a trusting and rewarding relationship with her.

Nurses in general hospitals may be called on, in different situations, to exercise their psychosocial skills. This case is one example.

EXAM QUESTIONS

CHAPTER 15
Questions 97–100

97. The nurse maintains competence in nursing is a provision from which of the following?

   a. ANA's Code for Nurses

   b. Patient's Bill of Rights

   c. Professional Practice Guidelines

   d. Standards of Practice for Psychiatric and Mental Health Nursing

98. Which of the following issues is *not* considered an ethical concern by Bandman and Bandman?

   a. Quality of life versus quantity of life

   b. Telling the truth versus telling a lie

   c. Freedom versus control

   d. Autonomy versus dependence

99. Which of the following are two current ethical issues in psychiatric nursing?

   a. Involuntary hospitalization and right to life

   b. Least restrictive alternative and right to die

   c. Informed consent and right to vote

   d. Least restrictive alternative and involuntary hospitalization

100. Which of the following is the legal concern addressed in the Tarasoff decision?

   a. Informed consent versus right to life

   b. Competency versus commitment

   c. Duty to warn versus confidentiality

   d. Privilege versus confidentiality

APPENDIX

NUMERIC LISTING OF DSM-IV DIAGNOSES AND CODES[1]

290.0   Dementia of the Alzheimer's type, with late onset, uncomplicated

    290.10   Dementia due to Creutzfeldt-Jakob disease

    290.10   Dementia due to Pick's disease

    290.10   Dementia of the Alzheimer's type, with early onset, uncomplicated

290.11   Dementia of the Alzheimer's type, with early onset, with delirium

290.12   Dementia of the Alzheimer's type, with early onset, with delusions

290.13   Dementia of the Alzheimer's type, with early onset, with depressed mood

290.20   Dementia of the Alzheimer's type, with late onset, with delusions

290.21   Dementia of the Alzheimer's type, with late onset, with depressed mood

290.3   Dementia of the Alzheimer's type, with late onset, with delirium

290.40   Vascular dementia, uncomplicated

290.41   Vascular dementia, with delirium

290.42   Vascular dementia, with delusions

290.43   Vascular dementia, with depressed mood

    291.0   Alcohol intoxication delirium

    291.0   Alcohol withdrawal delirium

291.1   Alcohol-induced persisting amnestic disorder

291.2   Alcohol-induced persisting dementia

291.3   Alcohol-induced psychotic disorder, with hallucinations

291.5   Alcohol-induced psychotic disorder, with delusions

291.8

    Alcohol-induced anxiety disorder

    Alcohol-induced mood disorder

    Alcohol-induced sexual dysfunction

    Alcohol-induced sleep disorder

    Alcohol withdrawal

291.9   Alcohol-related disorder NOS

292.0

    Amphetamine withdrawal

    Cocaine withdrawal

    Nicotine withdrawal

    Opioid withdrawal

    Other (or unknown) substance withdrawal

    Sedative, hypnotic, or anxiolytic withdrawal

292.11

    Amphetamine-induced psychotic disorder, with delusions

    Cannabis-induced psychotic disorder, with delusions

    Cocaine-induced psychotic disorder, with delusions

    Hallucinogen-induced psychotic disorder, with delusions

    Opioid-induced psychotic disorder, with delusions

    Other (or unknown) substance-induced psychotic disorder, with delusions

    Phencyclidine (PCP)-induced psychotic disorder, with delusions

    Sedative-, hypnotic-, or anxiolytic-induced

---

[1] To maintain compatibility with ICD-9-CM, some DSM-IV diagnoses share the same code numbers. These are indicated in this list by being indented.

Note: NOS = not otherwise specified.

Source: American Psychiatric Association. (1994). *Diagnostic and statistical manual of mental disorders* (4th ed.). Washington, DC: Author.

psychotic disorder, with delusions

292.12

Amphetamine-induced psychotic disorder, with hallucinations

Cannabis-induced psychotic disorder, with hallucinations

Cocaine-induced psychotic disorder, with hallucinations

Hallucinogen-induced psychotic disorder, with hallucinations

Inhalant-induced psychotic disorder, with hallucinations

Opioid-induced psychotic disorder, with hallucinations

Other (or unknown) substance-induced psychotic disorder, with hallucinations

292.81

Amphetamine intoxication delirium

Cannabis intoxication delirium

Cocaine intoxication delirium

Hallucinogen intoxication delirium

Inhalant intoxication delirium

Opioid intoxication delirium

Other (or unknown) substance-induced delirium

Phencyclidine intoxication delirium

Sedative, hypnotic, or anxiolytic intoxication delirium

Sedative, hypnotic, or anxiolytic withdrawal delirium

292.82

Inhalant-induced persisting dementia

Other (or unknown) substance-induced persisting dementia

Sedative-, hypnotic-, or anxiolytic-induced persisting dementia

292.83

Other (or unknown) substance-induced persisting amnestic disorder

Sedative-, hypnotic-, or anxiolytic-induced persisting amnestic disorder

292.84

Amphetamine-induced mood disorder

Cocaine-induced mood disorder

Hallucinogen-induced mood disorder

Inhalant-induced mood disorder

Opioid-induced mood disorder

Other (or unknown) substance-induced mood disorder

Phencyclidine-induced mood disorder

Sedative-, hypnotic-, or anxiolytic-induced mood disorder

292.89

Amphetamine-induced anxiety disorder

Amphetamine-induced sexual dysfunction

Amphetamine-induced sleep disorder

Amphetamine intoxication

Caffeine-induced anxiety disorder

Caffeine-induced sleep disorder

Cannabis-induced anxiety disorder

Cannabis intoxication

Cocaine-induced anxiety disorder

Cocaine-induced sexual dysfunction

Cocaine-induced sleep disorder

Cocaine intoxication

Hallucinogen-induced anxiety disorder

Hallucinogen intoxication

Hallucinogen persisting perception disorder

Inhalant-induced anxiety disorder

Inhalant intoxication

Opioid-induced sleep disorder

Opioid-induced sexual dysfunction

Opioid intoxication

Other (or unknown) substance-induced anxiety disorder

Other (or unknown) substance-induced sexual dysfunction

Other (or unknown) substance-induced sleep disorder

Other (or unknown) substance intoxication

Phencyclidine-induced anxiety disorder

Phencyclidine intoxication

Sedative-, hypnotic-, or anxiolytic-induced anxiety disorder

Sedative-, hypnotic-, or anxiolytic-induced sexual dysfunction

Sedative-, hypnotic-, or anxiolytic-induced sleep disorder

Sedative, hypnotic, or anxiolytic intoxication

292.9

Amphetamine-related disorder NOS

Caffeine-related disorder NOS

Cannabis-related disorder NOS

Cocaine-related disorder NOS

Hallucinogen-related disorder NOS

Inhalant-related disorder NOS

Nicotine-related disorder NOS

Opioid-related disorder NOS

Other (or unknown) substance-related disorder NOS

Phencyclidine-related disorder NOS

Sedative-, hypnotic,- or anxiolytic-related disorder NOS

293.00

Delirium due to…(indicate the general medical condition)

293.81 Psychotic disorder due to…(indicate the general medical condition) with delusions

293.82 Psychotic disorder due to…(indicate the general medical condition) with hallucinations

293.83 Mood disorder due to…(indicate the general medical condition)

293.89

Anxiety disorder due to…(indicate the general medical condition)

Catatonic disorder due to…(indicate the general medical condition)

293.9 Mental disorder NOS due to…(indicate the general medical condition)

294.8

Amnestic disorder due to…(indicate the general medical condition)

Dementia NOS

294.9

Cognitive disorder NOS

Dementia due to HIV disease

295.10 Schizophrenia, disorganized type

295.20 Schizophrenia, catatonic type

295.30 Schizophrenia, paranoid type

295.40 Schizophreniform disorder

295.60 Schizophrenia, residual type

295.70 Schizoaffective disorder

296.00 Bipolar I disorder, single manic episode, unspecified

296.01 Bipolar I disorder, single manic episode, mild

296.02 Bipolar I disorder, single manic episode, moderate

296.03 Bipolar I disorder, single manic episode, severe without psychotic features

296.04 Bipolar I disorder, single manic episode, severe with psychotic features

296.05 Bipolar I disorder, single manic episode, in partial remission

296.06 Bipolar I disorder, single manic episode, in full remission

296.20 Major depressive disorder, single episode, unspecified

296.21 Major depressive disorder, single episode, mild

296.22 Major depressive disorder, single episode, moderate

296.23 Major depressive disorder, single episode, severe, without psychotic features

296.24 Major depressive disorder, single episode, with psychotic features

296.25 Major depressive disorder, single episode, in partial remission

296.26 Major depressive disorder, single episode, in full remission

296.30 Major depressive disorder, recurrent, unspecified

296.31 Major depressive disorder, recurrent, mild

296.32 Major depressive disorder, recurrent, moderate

296.33 Major depressive disorder, recurrent, severe, with out psychotic features

296.34 Major depressive disorder, recurrent, severe, with psychotic features

296.35 Major depressive disorder, recurrent, in partial remission

296.36 Major depressive disorder, recurrent, in full remission

296.40

Bipolar I disorder, most recent episode hypomanic

Bipolar I disorder, most recent episode manic, unspecified

296.41 Bipolar I disorder, most recent episode manic, mild

296.42 Bipolar I disorder, manic, moderate

296.43 Bipolar I disorder, most recent episode manic, severe without psychotic features

296.44 Bipolar I disorder, most recent episode manic, severe with psychotic features

296.45 Bipolar I disorder, manic, in partial remission

296.46 Bipolar I disorder, manic, in full remission

296.50 Bipolar I disorder, most recent episode depressed, unspecified

296.51   Bipolar I disorder, most recent episode depressed, mild

296.52   Bipolar I disorder, most recent episode depressed, moderate

296.53   Bipolar I disorder, most recent episode depressed, severe, without psychotic features

296.54   Bipolar I disorder, most recent episode depressed, severe, with psychotic features

296.55   Bipolar I disorder, most recent episode depressed, in partial remission

296.56   Bipolar I disorder, most recent episode depressed, in full remission

296.60   Bipolar I disorder, most recent episode mixed, unspecified

296.61   Bipolar I disorder, most recent episode mixed, mild

296.62   Bipolar I disorder, most recent episode mixed, moderate

296.63   Bipolar I disorder, most recent episode mixed, severe, without psychotic features

296.64   Bipolar I disorder, most recent episode mixed, severe, with psychotic features

296.65   Bipolar I disorder, most recent episode mixed, in partial remission

296.66   Bipolar I disorder, most recent episode mixed, in full remission

296.7   Bipolar I disorder, most recent episode unspecified

296.80   Bipolar disorder NOS

296.90   Mood disorder NOS

297.1   Delusional disorder

297.3   Shared psychotic disorder

298.8   Brief psychotic disorder

298.9   Psychotic disorder NOS

299.00   Autistic disorder

299.80

   Asperger's disorder

   Pervasive developmental disorder NOS

   Rett's disorder

300.00   Anxiety disorder NOS

300.01   Panic disorder, without agoraphobia

300.02   Generalized anxiety disorder

300.11   Conversion disorder

300.12   Dissociative amnesia

300.13   Dissociative fugue

300.14   Dissociative identity disorder

300.15   Dissociative disorder NOS

300.16   Factitious disorder with predominantly psychological signs and symptoms

300.19

   Factitious disorder NOS

   Factitious disorder with combined psychological and physical signs and symptoms

   Factitious disorder with predominantly physical signs and symptoms

300.21   Panic disorder, with agoraphobia

300.22   Agoraphobia without history of panic disorder

300.23   Social phobia

300.29   Specific phobia

300.3   Obsessive-compulsive disorder

300.4   Dysthymic disorder

300.6   Depersonalization disorder

300.7   Body dysmorphic disorder

300.7   Hypochondriasis

    300.81   Somatization disorder

    300.81   Somatoform disorder NOS

    300.81   Undifferentiated somatoform disorder

300.9   Unspecified mental disorder (nonpsychotic)

301.0   Paranoid personality disorder

301.13   Cyclothymic disorder

301.20   Schizoid personality disorder

301.22   Schizotypal personality disorder

301.4   Obsessive-compulsive personality disorder

301.50   Histrionic personality disorder

301.6   Dependent personality disorder

301.7   Antisocial personality disorder

301.81   Narcissistic personality disorder

301.82   Avoidant personality disorder

301.83   Borderline personality disorder

301.9   Personality disorder NOS

302.2   Pedophilia

302.3   Transvestic fetishism

302.4   Exhibitionism

302.6   Gender identity disorder in children

302.6   Gender identity disorder NOS

302.70   Sexual dysfunction NOS

302.71   Hypoactive sexual desire disorder

    302.72   Female sexual arousal disorder

    302.72   Male erectile disorder

302.73   Female orgasmic disorder

302.74   Male orgasmic disorder

302.75   Premature ejaculation

302.76   Dyspareunia (not due to a general medical condition)

302.79   Sexual aversion disorder

302.81   Fetishism

302.82   Voyeurism

302.83   Sexual masochism

302.84   Sexual sadism

302.85   Gender identity disorder in adolescents or adults

302.89   Frotteurism

302.9   Paraphilia NOS

302.9   Sexual disorder NOS

303.00   Alcohol intoxication

303.90   Alcohol dependence

304.00   Opioid dependence

304.10   Sedative, hypnotic, or anxiolytic dependence

304.20   Cocaine dependence

304.30   Cannabis dependence

304.40   Amphetamine dependence

304.50   Hallucinogen dependence

304.60   Inhalant dependence

304.80   Polysubstance dependence

   304.90   Other (or unknown) substance dependence

   304.90   Phencyclidine dependence

305.00   Alcohol abuse

305.10   Nicotine dependence

305.20   Cannabis abuse

305.30   Hallucinogen abuse

305.40   Sedative, hypnotic, or anxiolytic abuse

305.50   Opioid abuse

305.60   Cocaine abuse

305.70   Amphetamine abuse

   305.90   Caffeine intoxication

   305.90   Inhalant abuse

   305.90   Other (or unknown) substance abuse

   305.90   Phencyclidine abuse

306.51   Vaginismus (not due to a general medical condition)

307.0   Stuttering

307.1   Anorexia nervosa

307.20   Tic disorder NOS

307.21   Transient tic disorder

307.22   Chronic motor or vocal tic disorder

307.23   Tourette's disorder

307.3   Stereotypic movement disorder

   307.42   Insomnia related to…(indicate the Axis I or Axis II disorder)

   307.42   Primary insomnia

   307.44   Hypersomnia related to…(indicate the Axis I or Axis II disorder)

   307.44   Primary hypersomnia

307.45   Circadian rhythm sleep disorder

   307.46   Sleep terror disorder

   307.46   Sleepwalking disorder

   307.47   Dyssomnia NOS

   307.47   Nightmare disorder

   307.47   Parasomnia NOS

307.50   Eating disorder NOS

307.51   Bulimia nervosa

307.52   Pica

307.53   Rumination disorder

307.59   Feeding disorder of infancy or early childhood

307.6   Enuresis (not due to a general medical condition)

307.7   Encopresis, without constipation and overflow incontinence

307.80   Pain disorder associated with psychological factors

307.89   Pain disorder associated with psychological factors and a general medical condition

307.9   Communication disorder NOS

308.3   Acute stress disorder

309.0   Adjustment disorder with depressed mood

309.21   Separation anxiety disorder

309.24   Adjustment disorder with anxiety

309.28   Adjustment disorder with mixed anxiety and depressed mood

309.3   Adjustment disorder with disturbance of conduct

309.4   Adjustment disorder with mixed disturbance of emotions and conduct

309.81   Posttraumatic stress disorder

309.9   Adjustment disorder unspecified

310.1   Personality change due to…(indicate the general medical condition)

311   Depressive disorder NOS

312.31   Pathologic gambling

312.32   Kleptomania

312.33   Pyromania

312.34   Intermittent explosive disorder

312.39 Trichotillomania

312.8 Conduct disorder

312.9 Disruptive behavior disorder NOS

313.23 Selective mutism

313.81 Oppositional defiant disorder

313.82 Identity problem

313.89 Reactive attachment disorder of infancy or early childhood

313.9 Disorder of infancy, childhood, or adolescence NOS

314.00 Attention-deficit/hyperactivity disorder, predominantly inattentive type

    314.01 Attention-deficit/hyperactivity disorder, combined type

    314.01 Attention-deficit/hyperactivity disorder, predominantly hyperactive-impulsive type

314.9 Attention-deficit/hyperactivity disorder, NOS

315.00 Reading disorder

315.1 Mathematics disorder

315.2 Disorder of written expression

    315.31 Expressive language disorder

    315.31 Mixed receptive-expressive language disorder

315.39 Phonologic disorder

315.4 Developmental coordination disorder

315.9 Learning disorder NOS

316 …(specified psychological factor) affecting… (indicate the general medical condition)

317 Mild mental retardation

318.0 Moderate mental retardation

318.1 Severe mental retardation

318.2 Profound mental retardation

319 Mental retardation, severity unspecified

332.1 Neuroleptic-induced parkinsonism

333.1 Medication-induced postural tremor

333.7 Neuroleptic-induced acute dystonia

333.82 Neuroleptic-induced tardive dyskinesia

333.90 Medication-induced movement disorder NOS

333.92 Neuroleptic malignant syndrome

333.99 Neuroleptic-induced acute akathisia

347 Narcolepsy

607.84 Male erectile disorder due to…(indicate the general medical condition)

608.89 Male dyspareunia due to…(indicate the general medical condition)

608.89 Male hypoactive sexual desire disorder due to…(indicate the general medical condition)

608.89 Other male sexual dysfunction due to…(indicate the general medical condition)

625.0 Female dyspareunia due to…(indicate the general medical condition)

    625.8 Female hypoactive sexual desire disorder due to…(indicate the general medical condition)

    625.8 Other female sexual dysfunction due to…(indicate the general medical condition)

780.09 Delirium NOS

780.52 Sleep disorder due to…(indicate the general medical condition), insomnia type

780.54 Sleep disorder due to…(indicate the general medical condition), hypersomnia type

    780.59 Breathing-related sleep disorder

    780.59 Sleep disorder due to…(indicate the general medical condition), mixed type

    780.59 Sleep disorder due to…(indicate the general medical condition), parasomnia type

780.9 Age-related cognitive decline

787.6 Encopresis, with constipation and overflow incontinence

    799.9 Diagnosis deferred on Axis II

    799.9 Diagnosis or condition deferred on Axis I

995.2 Adverse effects of medication NOS

    995.5 Neglect of child (if focus of attention is on victim)

    995.5 Physical abuse of child (if focus of attention is on victim)

    995.5 Sexual abuse of child (if focus of attention is on victim)

    995.81 Physical abuse of adult (if focus of attention is on victim)

    995.81 Sexual abuse of adult (if focus of attention is on victim)

V15.81 Noncompliance with treatment

    V61.1 Partner relational problem

    V61.1 Physical abuse of adult

    V61.1 Sexual abuse of adult

V61.20 Parent-child relational problem

V61.21   Neglect of child

V61.21   Physical abuse of child

V61.21   Sexual abuse of child

V61.8   Sibling relational problem

V61.9   Relational problem related to a mental disorder or general medical condition

V62.2   Occupational problem

V62.3   Academic problem

V62.4   Acculturation problem

V62.81   Relational problem NOS

V62.82   Bereavement

V62.89   Borderline intellectual functioning

V62.89   Phase of life problem

V62.89   Religious or spiritual problem

V65.2   Malingering

V71.01   Adult antisocial behavior

V71.02   Childhood or adolescent antisocial behavior

V71.09   No diagnosis on Axis II

V71.09   No diagnosis or condition on Axis I

GLOSSARY

Acuity: Intensity of illness, stated as high acuity or low acuity; may refer to an individual's illness, or to the state of many patients within the milieu (i.e., a milieu with high acuity).

Affect: The facial expression and body language that relfect or indicate an emotion.

Akathisia: Motor restlessness as caused by the side effect of antipsychotic medications (major tranquilizers); often described by patients as an inability to sit still or to keep one's legs still; may be mistakenly assessed as anxiety or insomnia, because akathisia prevents lying still long enough to fall asleep.

Alcoholism: A disorder characterized by out-of-control consumption of alcohol, resulting in biological, social, and vocational functional impairment.

Aliphatics: A subclass of the phenothiazines; includes chlorpromazine, promazine, and tri-flupromazine.

Amnestic disorder: A disorder characterized by severe impairment of both short- and long-term memory; usually with organic cause; may be psychogenic amnesia after stressful or conflict-ual events.

Anhedonia: An impairment in the ability to experience pleasure; often accompanies depression.

Anorexia: A loss of, or decrease in, appetite.

Anorexia nervosa: An eating disorder in which the person affected is severely preoccupied with food, dieting, and body image; characterized by failure to maintain normal body weight while misperceiving one's body as "fat"; using laxatives, diuretics, and self-induced vomiting to lose weight; may be so severe as to lead to death.

Anticholinergic side effects: A group of side effects that may occur with antipsychotic and antidepressant medications; includes dry mouth, constipation, blurred vision, urinary retention, mydriasis; more severe anticholinergic side effects may include agitation, confusion, hallucinations, and seizures.

Antidepressants: Medications with a primary indication for the relief of depression; major categories of antidepressants include the tricyclic antidepressants (TCAs), the monoamine oxidase inhibitors (MAOIs), the selective serotonin reuptake inhibitors (SSRIs), and the second-generation antidepressants.

Antipsychotics: Class of medications used for the alleviation of impaired thought processes (e.g., hallucinations, delusions) and/or a state of agitation; also referred to as major tranquilizers.

Anxiety: An emotional state, which may be a disorder in itself, a component of another emotional disorder (e.g., depression may be accompanied by anxiety), or an indication of a physical disorder (e.g., may accompany hypertension), characterized by internal restlessness, nervousness, and an inability to relax; may be of variable degrees of intensity; often rated on a scale of 1 to 4+, with 4+ being the most intense level of anxiety.

Anxiety disorders: A group of disorders characterized primarily by anxiety; includes panic disorder, obsessive-compulsive disorder, generalized anxiety disorder, phobic disorders, and posttraumatic stress disorder.

Anxiolytics: A class of medications used for the alleviation of signs and symptoms of anxiety or for the treatment of anxiety disorders; benzodiazepines fall within this class of medications.

Atypical depression: A depressive disorder, characterized by signs and symptoms of depression (*see* depressed affective disorder) and accompanied by excessive anxiety.

Benzodiazepines: A class of antianxiety medications with the intended effect of relief of anxiety; intended for short-term use, because long-term use may lead to dependence and require medically monitored withdrawal; some medications in this class are also intended for use with alcohol withdrawal, insomnia, muscle relaxation, and/or treatment of panic disorders.

Bipolar affective illness: A major mental illness characterized by episodes of mania and depression; usually diagnosed when the affected person is in his or her twenties; frequency of episodes of mania or depression vary from patient to patient; treatment of choice is with mood-stabilizing medications, such as lithium carbonate.

Borderline personality disorder: A personality disorder; may be seen with severe impairment in interpersonal relatedness and vocational functioning; characterized by emotional lability, reckless impulsiveness, inability to modulate anger, chronic feelings of emptiness or boredom, ineffective coping abilities, and recurrent suicidal thoughts or behaviors.

Bulimia nervosa: An eating disorder characterized by uncontrolled eating of excessive amounts of food, which is often followed by feelings of guilt, self-hate, or depression; often accompanied by the use of laxatives or self-induced vomiting to counter the binge eating.

Butyrophenones: Chemical class of antipsychotic medications; includes haloperidol.

Cognitive abilities: A person's abilities of thinking, including the ability to reason, to make inferences, and to understand.

Command hallucination: An auditory hallucination (*see* hallucinations) in which one or more voices instruct the affected person to act in a certain way; often a command that is dangerous to the person (e.g., jump off a bridge, walk in front of the car); the person who experiences the commands does not perceive any control over his or her response to them.

Competency: Mental competency; refers to a person's ability to think clearly, to display insight into the current situation, and to make sound judgments; in a legal sense, a person is assumed to be competent unless deemed incompetent by a court of law.

Concrete thinking: A lack of abstract thinking, seeing only the "night and day" of a situation, without the ability to go beyond to see the implied meaning, or more abstract meaning; making literal versus figurative interpretations of words or phrases.

Coping ability: The skill or ability to manage the various challenges that occur as a regular part of a person's life; may be assessed for a person or for a family unit.

Cyclothymic affective illness: A mild form of bipolar affective illness (*see* bipolar affective illness).

Delirium: A disordered mental status characterized by confusion, agitation, hallucinations; has various physical or mental causes.

Delirium tremens: A disordered mental state, or delirium, that occurs during withdrawal from alcohol; characterized by tremors, confusion, agitation, hallucinations, apprehension, and elevated vital signs; can lead to a medical emergency if not treated aggressively and in a timely manner.

Delusion: A false belief as a manifestation of a thought disorder; may be of various types, including paranoid, persecutory, religious, grandiose, nihilistic, and self-deprecatory.

Dementia: A progressive deterioration of the brain, of an organic nature; more than 50% of patients who have dementia have Alzheimer's disease; multi-infarct dementia and HIV dementia are other leading types; may cause variable degrees of impairment.

Depressed affective illness: Referred to as major depression; may be a single episode or a recurring illness; often characterized by vegetative signs and symptoms (loss of appetite, insomnia or hypersomnia, decreased ability to concentrate, decreased libido), hopelessness or helplessness, sadness, anhedonia, agitation, withdrawal, negativity, and suicidal ideations and behaviors.

Dihydroindolones: A class of antipsychotic medications; includes molindone.

Diphenylbutylpiperidines: A class of antipsychotic medications; includes pimozide.

DSM-IV: Acronym for the 1994 edition of *Diagnostic and Statistical Manual of Mental Disorders* published by the American Psychiatric Association; describes the mental disorders and the specific criteria needed to make a definitive diagnosis.

Duty to warn: A group of statutes related to professional responsibilities to warn intended victims of a patient's statements of intent to harm; the most famous comes from the *Tarasoff v. Regents of University of California* case.

Dyskinesias: Movement disorders characterized by difficulty of movement or involuntary movement.

Dysthymic affective illness: A mood disorder similar to depression, with chronic versus episodic signs and symptoms and general, overall unhappiness; often results in impairments in interpersonal and vocational functioning.

Echolalia: Behavior in which the person affected automatically repeats what is said to him or her; may be present with a psychotic disorder.

Euphoria: An emotional state of elation; as a component of mental illness, a state dramatically out of perspective with the person's current situation.

Extrapyramidal side effects: A group of side effects of the antipsychotics (major tranquilizers); more common with the higher potency ones; includes akathisia, pseudoparkinsonism, acute dystonic reactions, and tardive dyskinesia; named for the area of the brain involved.

Flight of ideas: An alteration in thought processes characterized by the jumping from one idea to another unrelated idea, usually in rapid succession; often accompanies the manic phase of bipolar affective disorder.

Grandiosity: An alteration in thought processes in which the affected person has delusional beliefs that he or she is of great importance or has superhuman abilities (e.g., the person may believe that he or she holds the key to world peace, or that he or she can fly like the birds).

Hallucination: A perceptual disorder, as a manifestation of a thought disorder, in which the person affected experiences sensations that are not present by other people's perceptions; as a manifestation of a thought disorder, these are usually auditory; may be visual, tactile, gustatory, or olfactory, but these are more often a manifestation of an organic disorder.

Histrionic personality disorder: A personality disorder characterized by a constant need for approval, an exaggerated expression of emotion, a discomfort with not being the center of attention, and self-centeredness.

Hyperreligiosity: An abnormally high focus on religious ideas and beliefs; as a component of an emotional illness, often of a delusional nature.

Hypersexuality: An abnormally high libido and focus on sexual thoughts as may accompany some psychiatric illnesses (e.g., the manic phase of bipolar affective illness).

Inappropriate affect: Facial expression or body language that is incongruent with the content of thought, mood, or emotion.

Insight: Awareness of one's situation and the factors affecting the situation; a lack of insight may accompany emotional disorders and compromise a person's ability to make appropriate decisions and use good, sound judgment.

Lethargy: A psychobiological state in which the affected person has little energy, little interest or desire to mobilize his or her energies; sluggishness.

Lithium carbonate: A mood-stabilizing medication.

Looseness of association: An alteration in thought processes in which the affected person's speech reflects a lack of organized, sensible connectedness between subjects; for example, when talking of feeling blue, jumping to the subject of the blue sky.

Manic affective illness: *See* bipolar affective illness.

Manipulate: To get one's needs met indirectly, often at the expense of others, and often when a more direct expression of one's needs would be unsuccessful in achieving the desired result.

Mental status examination: A comprehensive examination of a person's emotional state and thinking processes; when used in making a diagnosis of a psychiatric illness, the equivalent of a physical examination in making a physical diagnosis.

Monoamine oxidase inhibitors (MAOIs): A class of antidepressant medications that work by inhibiting monoamine oxidase in the synaptic cleft; includes Nardil, Parnate, Marplan; patients taking these medications must follow a strict diet (no foods containing the amino acid tyramine) and should check with their physician before taking any over-the-counter medications; failure to follow the diet and medication restrictions could result in a hypertensive crisis.

Mood: A person's emotion that colors his or her perception of the world and people around him or her.

Mutism: Voicelessness with an emotional cause rather than a physical cause.

Neuroleptics: Medications that affect the brain and nervous system.

Noncompliance: Failure to follow the prescribed treatment regimen.

Obsessive-compulsive disorder: A psychiatric disorder characterized by recurrent obsessional thinking and recurrent compulsive behaviors severe enough to interfere with normal interpersonal and vocational functioning.

Organic anxiety disorder: An organic disorder characterized by recurrent panic attacks or by generalized anxiety.

Organic delusional disorder: An organic disorder characterized by alteration in thought processes in which the person affected has false beliefs (*see* delusions); most often caused by use of drugs such as amphetamines, cannabis, and hallucinogens.

Organic hallucinosis: An organic disorder characterized by alteration in thought processes in which the person affected has hallucinations; most often caused by chronic alcohol or drug abuse.

Organic mood disorder: An organic disorder characterized by mood disturbances, either of depression or mania.

Organic personality syndrome: An organic disorder characterized by marked changes in a person's personality; most often caused by head trauma or brain injury.

Orthostatic hypotension: A sudden drop in blood pressure that occurs when a person changes position (e.g., changes from lying down to sitting or standing); often a side effect of use of some of the psychotropic medications.

Panic: An episode of severe anxiety in which the person affected experiences fearfulness, apprehension, foreboding, diaphoresis, elevated vital signs, and changes in psychomotor activity along with the perception that if relief is not promptly obtained, the person will experience an unfortunate fate (e.g., "going crazy" or "dying"); may be a single episode or recurring episodes.

Phenothiazines: A major class of antipsychotic medications; includes aliphatics, piperidines, and piperazines.

Piperidines: A subclass of the phenothiazines; includes thioridazine and mesoridazine.

Piperazines: A subclass of the phenothiazines; includes fluphenazine, trifluoperazine, and perphenazine.

Psychiatric: Pertaining to a person's emotional state and thought functioning.

Psychomotor retardation: A dramatic decrease in a person's physical activity, as may accompany severe depression.

Psychosis: A disordered state of thinking, often characterized by hallucinations or delusions; has a variety of causes; may be acute or an ongoing part of a persistent mental disorder.

Psychosocial: Pertaining to those aspects of a person that are of psychological or social origins.

Psychopharmacological: Pertaining to medications that have intended effects on a person's emotional state or thought processes.

Recurrent major depression: Episodes of major depression (*see* depressive affective disorder) that occur more than once; may recur one time or several times over many years.

Regression: A return to an earlier stage of development; a mental mechanism used to resolve conflict by returning to a behavior that was more successful in having one's needs met.

Schizophrenia: A severe and persistent mental illness characterized by disordered thinking, impaired social and vocational functioning; the most disabling of the mental illnesses.

Somatic: Pertaining to the body; somatic signs and symptoms of emotional or mental disorders may include decreased appetite, insomnia, gastrointestinal distress, decreased libido, and decreased ability to concentrate.

Splitting: A defensive mechanism in which a person sees most objects as either good or bad and cannot distinguish the "gray," seeing only in "black or white"; the person often behaves in a manner that reinforces this way of viewing others and the world (e.g., a patient identifies a particular staff member as "the only one who truly understands me" and all others as "they don't care for me like you do," thereby working members of the staff against each other or "splitting" their cohesiveness and therefore their effectiveness in helping the person).

Tangential speech: A pattern of speech in which a person strays from the subject at hand, going off into related topics that have no relevance to the current discussion.

Tardive dyskinesia: A movement disorder as an adverse effect of long-term use (at least 6 months) of antipsychotics (major tranquilizers); characterized by involuntary, choreathetoid movements of the upper extremities and facial muscles; may become severely disabling.

Therapeutic relationships: Helping relationships between a patient and a mental health professional in which the "therapeutic use of self" principle is combined with the behavioral and psychosocial sciences to assist the patient on the road to recovery; relationship falls within strict ethical boundaries.

Thioxanthenes: A class of antipsychotic medications; includes chlorprothixene and thiothixene.

Thought content: The subject focus of a person's thinking; in psychiatric assessments, thought content that is negativistic, fearful, lonely, suspicious, and so forth may be clues to emotional or mental disorders.

BIBLIOGRAPHY

Aguilera, D. C. (1990). *Crisis intervention: Theory and methodology* (6th ed). St. Louis: Mosby.

American Hospital Association. (1992). *A patient's bill of rights.* Chicago: Author.

American Nurses Association. (1985). *Code for nurses.* Kansas City, MO: Author.

American Nurses Association. (1994). *Standards of psychiatric and mental health nursing practice.* Kansas City, MO: Author.

American Psychiatric Association. (1994). *Diagnostic and statistical manual of mental disorders* (4th ed.). Washington, DC: Author.

Bandman, E. L., & Bandman, B. (1990). *Nursing ethics through the life span* (2nd ed.). East Norwalk, CT: Appleton & Lange.

Barry, P. D. (1989). *Psychosocial nursing assessment intervention* (2nd ed.). Philadelphia: Lippincott.

Beck, A. T. (1967). *Depression: Clinical, experimental and theoretical aspects.* New York: Harper & Row.

Beck, A. T. (1976). *Cognitive therapy and the emotional disorders.* New York: International Universities Press.

Bell, C., et. al. (1994). Response of emergency rooms to victims of interpersonal violence. *Hospital and Community Psychiatry, 45*(2).

Bennett, E. G., & Woolf, D. (1991). *Substance abuse* (2nd ed.). Albany, NY: Delmar Publishing.

Blair, D. T., & Dauner, A. (1993). Neuroleptic malignant syndrome: Liability in nursing practice. *Journal of Psychosocial Nursing, 31*(2).

Blair, D. T., & New, S. A. (1991). Assaultive behavior: Know the risks. *Journal of Psychosocial Nursing, 29*(11).

Borders, C. (Sr. Ed.). (1985–1986). A Patient Care roundtable with patients who had coronary bypass surgery. *Patient Care.*

Burckhardt, C. S. (1986). Ethical issues in compliance. *Topics in Clinical Nursing, 7*(4), 9–16.

Burgess, A. W. (1990). *Psychiatric nursing in the hospital and community* (5th ed.). East Norwalk, CT: Appleton & Lange.

Campbell, R. J. (1989). *Psychiatric dictionary* (6th ed.). New York: Oxford University Press.

Carroll-Johnson, R. M., & Paquette, M. (1994). *Classification of nursing diagnoses: Proceedings of the tenth conference: North American Nursing Diagnosis Association.* Philadelphia: Lippincott.

Chapman, T. (1991). The nurse's role in neuroleptic medications. *Journal of Psychosocial Nursing, 29*(6).

Cheng-Chung, C., et al. (1991). A follow-up of patients with neuroleptic malignant syndrome. *Hospital and Community Psychiatry, 42*(2).

Chitty, K. K., & Maynard, C. K. (1986). Managing manipulation. *Journal of Psychosocial Nursing, 24,* 9–13.

Clark, S. R. (1986). Compliance and health behaviors. *Topics in Clinical Nursing, 7*(4), 39–46.

Corcoran, D. K. (1988). Helping patients who've had near-death experiences. *Nursing 88, 11,* 34–39.

Courage, M. M., et al. (1993). Suicide in the elderly: Staying in control. *Journal of Psychosocial Nursing, 31*(7).

Critchley, D. L., & Maurin, J. T. (Eds.). (1985). *The clinical specialist in psychiatric mental health nursing.* New York: Wiley.

Cummings, K. M., Becker, M. H., Kirscht, J. P., & Levin, N. W. (1982). Psychosocial factors affecting adherence to medical regimens in a group of hemodialysis patients. *Medical Care, 20,* 567–580.

Cummings, K. M., Becker, M. H., Kirscht, J. P., & Levin, N. W. (1984). Construct validity comparisons of three methods for measuring patient compliance. *Health Services Research, 19*(1), 103–115.

Curtin, S. L. (1993). Recognizing multiple personality disorder. *Journal of Psychosocial Nursing, 31*(2).

Deering, C. G. (1987). Developing a therapeutic alliance with the anorexia nervosa client. *Journal of Psychosocial Nursing, 25*(3).

DeLaune, S.C. (1991). Effective limit setting: How to avoid being manipulated. *Nursing Clinics of North America, 26*(3).

Dellasega, C. (1991). Meeting the mental health needs of elderly clients. *Journal of Psychosocial Nursing, 29*(2).

Dillon, N. B. (1992). Screening system for tardive dyskinesia: Development and implementation. *Journal of Psychosocial Nursing, 30*(10).

Donovan, J. L., & Blake, D. R. (1992). Patient noncompliance: Deviance or reasoned decision making. *Social Science Medicine, 34*(5).

Drew, N. (1991). Combating the social isolation of chronic mental illness. *Journal of Psychosocial Nursing, 29*(6).

Drug handbook. (1993). Springhouse, PA: Springhouse Corp.

Edel, M. K. (1985). Noncompliance: An appropriate diagnosis? *Nursing Outlook, 33*(4), 183–185.

Ellis, N. K. (1988). Manipulation. In C. K. Beck, R. P. Rawlins, & S. R. Williams (Eds.), *Mental health-psychiatric nursing: A holistic life-cycle approach* (pp. 415–428). St. Louis: Mosby.

Feldmann, T. B. (1989). Legal issues in psychiatry. In *Manual of psychosocial nursing interventions* (pp. 293–298). Philadelphia: Saunders.

Fernandez, T. (1986). Classic: How to deal with overt aggression. *Issues in Mental Health Nursing, 8,* 79–83.

Field, W. E., Jr. (1988). Physical causes of depression. *Journal of Psychosocial Nursing, 23*(2).

Forman, L. (1993). Medication: Reasons and interventions for noncompliance. *Journal of Psychosocial Nursing, 31*(10).

Friedman, M., & Rosenman, R. (1974). *Type A behavior and your heart.* New York: Knopf.

Garritson, S. H. (1983). Degrees of restrictiveness. *Journal of Psychosocial Nursing, 21,* 17–23.

Groves, J. E. (1978). Taking care of the hateful patient. *New England Journal of Medicine, 298,* 883–887.

Hackett, T. P., & Stern, T. A. (1987). Suicide and other disruptive states. In T. P. Hackett & N. H. Cassem (Eds.), *Massachusetts General Hospital: Handbook of general hospital psychiatry* (pp. 268–296). Littleton, MA: PSG Publishing.

Hofland, S. L., & Dardis, P. O. (1992). Bulimia nervosa: Associated physical problems. *Journal of Psychosocial Nursing, 30*(2).

Hradek, E. (1988). Crisis intervention and suicide. *Journal of Psychosocial Nursing, 26,* 24–27.

Jones, M. K. (1988). Patient violence. *Journal of Psychosocial Nursing, 26,* 12–17.

Junginger, J. (1995, September). Command hallucinations and the prediction of dangerousness. *Psychiatric Services.*

Kaplan, H. I., & Sadock, B. J. (1991). *Synopsis of psychiatry: Behavioral sciences clinical psychiatry* (6th ed.). Baltimore: Williams & Wilkins.

Keltner, N., et al. (1991). *Psychiatric nursing: A psychotherapeutic approach.* St. Louis: Mosby–Year Book.

Kerr, N. J. (1988). Depression. *Perspectives in Psychiatric Care, 24,* 48–53.

King, K. (1990). Strategies for enhancing compliance in the dialysis elderly. *American Journal of Kidney Diseases, 15,* 351–353.

Kirsta, A. (1986). *The book of stress survival.* New York: Simon and Schuster.

Krishel, S., & Jackimczyk, K. (1991, February). Cyclic antidepressants, lithium and neuroleptic agents. *Psychiatric Aspects of Emergency Medicine.*

Kumler, F. R. (1963). The interpersonal interpretation of manipulation. In S. F. Burd & M. S. Marshall (Eds.), *Some clinical approaches to psychiatric nursing.* New York: Macmillan.

Laben, J. K., & MacLean, C. P. (1989). *Legal issues and guidelines for nurses who care for the mentally ill* (2nd ed.). Owings Mills, MD: National Health Publications.

Lobl, J., & Carbone, L. (1992, January). Emergency management of cocaine intoxication. *Postgraduate Medicine.*

McCord, M. A. (1986). Compliance: Self-care or compromise? *Topics in Clinical Nursing, 7*(4), 1–8.

McFarland, G., & Thomas, M. D. (1991). *Psychiatric mental health nursing: Application of the nursing process.* Philadelphia: Lippincott.

McGurn, W. C. (1981). *People with cardiac problems: Nursing concepts.* Philadelphia: Lippincott.

McMorrow, M. E. (1981). The manipulative patient. *American Journal of Nursing, 81,* 1188–1191.

McNiel, D. E., & Binder, R. L. (1994). The relationship between acute psychiatric symptoms, diagnosis, and short-term risk of violence. *Hospital and Community Psychiatry, 45*(2).

McShane, R., et al. (1994). Psychological distress in family members living with human immunodeficiency virus/acquired immune deficiency syndrome. *Archives of Psychiatric Nursing, 8*(1).

Mellick, E., et al. (1992). Suicide among elderly white men: Development of a profile. *Journal of Psychosocial Nursing, 30*(2).

Montgomery, P., & Johnson, B. (1992). The stress of marriage to an alcoholic. *Journal of Psychosocial Nursing, 30*(10).

Mound, B., et al. (1991). The expanded role of nurse case managers. *Journal of Psychosocial Nursing, 29*(6).

Murray, R. B., & Huelskoetter, M. M. W. (1983). *Psychiatric/mental health nursing: Giving emotional care.* Englewood Cliffs, NJ: Prentice-Hall.

Nadler-Moodie, M. (1986). The multiple roles of psychiatric nurses. In A. H. Collins & H. K. Krauss (Eds.), *The provider's guide to hospital-based psychiatric services* (pp. 309–326). Rockville, MD: Aspen.

North American Nursing Diagnosis Association. (1994). *Nursing diagnoses: Definitions and classification, 1995–96.* Philadelphia: Author.

Padrick, K. P. (1986). Compliance: Myths and motivators. *Topics in Clinical Nursing, 7*(4), 17–22.

Peplau, H. E. (1952). *Interpersonal relations in nursing.* New York: Putnam.

Pomerantz, A. S., & de Nesnera, A. (1991). Informed consent, competency, and the illusion of rationality. *General Hospital Psychiatry, 13,* 138–142.

Puntil, C. (1991). Integrating three approaches to counter resistance in a noncompliant elderly client. *Journal of Psychosocial Nursing, 29*(2).

Rawlins, R. P., & Heacock, P. E. (1988). *The clinical manual of psychiatric nursing.* St. Louis: Mosby.

Regan-Kubinski, M. J., & Sharts-Engel. (1992). The HIV-infected woman: Illness cognition assessment. *Journal of Psychosocial Nursing, 30*(2).

Roberts, A. R. (1990). *Crisis intervention handbook.* Belmont, CA: Wadsworth.

Rosenbluth, M., et al. (1995, September). Suicide: The interaction of clinical and ethical issues. *Psychiatric Services.*

Rosner, R. (1986). Approaches to mental health and the law in the general hospital setting. In A. H. Collins & H. K. Krauss (Eds.), *The provider's guide to hospital-based psychiatric services.* Rockville, MD: Aspen.

Selye, H. (1976). *The stress of life* (rev. ed.). New York: McGraw-Hill.

Small, S. M. (1984). *A guide for psychiatric examination.* East Hanover, NJ: Sandoz.

Smith, M., & Buckwalter, K. C. (1992). Medication management, antidepressant drugs, and the elderly: An overview. *Journal of Psychosocial Nursing, 30*(10).

Snyder, M. S. (1984). Legal issues in psychiatric nursing. In S. Lego (Ed.), *The American handbook of psychiatric nursing.* Philadelphia: Lippincott.

Spratto, G. R., & Woods, A. L. (1995). *Nurse's drug reference 95.* Albany, NY: Delmar Publishing.

Strome, T. M. (1988). Restraining the elderly. *Journal of Psychosocial Nursing, 26,* 18–21.

Stuart, G. W. (1995). *Pocket guide to psychiatric nursing.* St. Louis: Mosby.

Stuart, G. W., & Sundeen, S. J. (1990). *Principles and practice of psychiatric nursing* (4th ed.). St. Louis: Mosby –Year Book.

Thompson, L. (1986). Peplau's theory: An application to short-term individual therapy. *Journal of Psychosocial Nursing, 24,* 26–31.

Thorne, S. E. (1990). Constructive noncompliance in chronic illness. *Holistic Nursing Practice, 5*(1), 62–69.

Townsend, M. C. (1988). *Nursing diagnoses in psychiatric nursing.* Philadelphia: Davis.

Trudeau, M. E. (1993). Informed consent: The patient's right to decide. *Journal of Psychosocial Nursing, 31*(6).

Ugarriza, D. N., & Gray, T. (1993). Alzheimer's disease: Nursing interventions for clients and caretakers. *Journal of Psychosocial Nursing, 31*(10).

U.S. Department of Health and Human Services, Public Health Service, Agency for Health Care Policy and Research. (1993). Depression in primary care: Detection, diagnosis, and treatment. *Journal of Psychosocial Nursing, 31*(6).

Welch-McCaffrey, D. (1986). To teach or not to teach? Overcoming barriers to patient education in geriatric oncology. *Oncology Nursing Forum, 13*(4), 25–30.

Whitley, G. (1991). Noncompliance. In G. K. McFarland & M. D. Thomas (Eds.), *Psychiatric mental health nursing: Application of the nursing process* (pp. 307–312). Philadelphia: Lippincott.

Wiley, P. L. (1968). Manipulation. In L. T. Zderad & H. C. Belcher (Eds.), *Developing behavioral concepts in nursing.*

Williams-Burgess, C., & Kimball, M. J. (1992). The neglected elder: A family systems approach. *Journal of Psychosocial Nursing, 30*(10).

Wilson, H. S., & Kneisl, C. R. (1992). *Psychiatric nursing* (4th ed.). Menlo Park, CA: Addison-Wesley.

Wing, D. M., & Hammer-Higgins, P. (1993). Determinants of denial: A study of alcoholics. *Journal of Psychosocial Nursing, 31*(2).

Wurzbach, M. E. (1991). The dilemma of withholding or withdrawing nutrition. Image: The *Journal of Nursing Scholarship, 22,* 226–230.

Young, M. S. (1986). Strategies for improving compliance. *Topics in Clinical Nursing, 7*(4), 31–38.

INDEX

PRETEST KEY

1.	D	Chapter 1
2.	D	Chapter 1
3.	D	Chapter 2
4.	A	Chapter 2
5.	D	Chapter 3
6.	C	Chapter 3
7.	D	Chapter 3
8.	D	Chapter 3
9.	C	Chapter 4
10.	C	Chapter 5
11.	D	Chapter 5
12.	A	Chapter 6
13.	C	Chapter 7
14.	C	Chapter 7
15.	A	Chapter 7
16.	B	Chapter 8
17.	C	Chapter 8
18.	D	Chapter 9
19.	A	Chapter 10
20.	B	Chapter 11
21.	D	Chapter 11
22.	D	Chapter 12
23.	B	Chapter 14
24.	D	Chapter 14
25.	C	Chapter 15

NOTES

NOTES

NOTES

NOTES

NOTES

NOTES